FLESHING OUT THE BONES

Case Histories
In The Practice
Of Chinese Medicine

BY CHARLES CHACE

Blue Poppy Press

Published by:

BLUE POPPY PRESS
1775 LINDEN AVE.
BOULDER, CO 80304

SECOND EDITION
NOVEMBER 1993

Library of Congress #91-076855
ISBN 0-936185-30-9

Printed at Westview Press, Boulder, CO
Cover printed at D & K Printing, Boulder, CO
Marbled paper for cover art courtesy of Christine J. Covert

This book is printed on archive quality, acid free, recycled paper.

10 9 8 7 6 5 4 3 2

ACKNOWLEDGMENTS

I would like to thank my friend and mentor Zhang Ting-liang for his help in clarifying many obscure passages of Chinese over the years. His assistance on this project has been of inestimable value. I am also indebted to Bob Flaws, an elder brother in my study of Chinese medicine, and Bob Felt, a crazy uncle. This volume is at least in part a result of the encouragement, support, and occasional kicks in the pants they have provided. Finally, I would like to thank Honora Wolfe for her editorial patience and forbearance.

CONTENTS

INTRODUCTION

Fleshing Out The Bones: Case Histories in the Practice of Chinese Medicine.

It is strange how seemingly trivial events can shape one's personal outlook in profound ways. Ten years ago an evening spent chatting with friends dramatically changed the way I thought about the use of Chinese medical literature in the study and practice of Traditional Chinese Medicine. One of the people present had recently returned from Taiwan and had begun practicing Chinese medicine in the area. This person spent a good part of the evening describing a variety of difficult cases she was currently seeing and researching in the case history literature. This came as something of a revelation to me. Up until that evening it hadn't really occurred to me that case histories were an essential part of doing one's clinical homework. This was largely because there were few, if any case histories available in English at the time. While it seems that little has changed since then, my appreciation for the case history literature of Chinese medicine has continued to grow.

Until now, efforts at translating the vast corpus of Chinese medicine literature into Western languages have focused largely on two fronts. The first is the translation of the premodern classics which conprise both the theoretical and therapeutic foundations of current TCM practice. Paul Unschuld's translation of the *Nan Jing* is perhaps the benchmark example of this genre. The second is the translation and/or complitaion of modern TCM textbooks such as *Fundamentals of Chinese Medicine* by Wiseman *et al.,* and Bensky and Barolet's *Chinese Herbal Medicine: Formulas and Strategies.* It should be frustratingly evident to any clinician that resources in these areas are scarce to say the least. Since it is difficult, if not impossible, to practice Traditional Chinese Medicine without these two types of literature, it is understandable why the few translators working in the field of Chinese medicine have chosen to begin with texts such as these.

Pre-modern classics such as the *Nei Jing, Nan Jing, Jin Gui Yao Lue,* and *Shang Han Lun* comprise the skeletal system of Chinese medicine. The concepts fundamental to the modern practice of Chinese medicine, known today as TCM, have their origins in these seminal works. They are the bare bones which give Chinese medicine, in all its permutations, its overall form. Contemporary textbooks present a modern synthesis of this information. There is often some misundertanding, however, as to the scope and limitations of these two genres of medical writing which have been and remain primarily teaching tools at the professional entry level.

While a few of the major premodern Chinese medical classics are now available in English, there is as yet a wealth of untapped information to be gleaned from premodern sources, significant pieces of useful material to be brought to the light of modern practice. Premodern sources do, however, present a number of difficulties to the busy clinician endeavoring to access them. In addition to the gemlike insights, which are the cornerstones of Chinese medical practice, they also contain ideas which have been left by the wayside because they did not pan out in clinical usage over the centuries. Therefore, it often takes some weeding to unearth the most useful information. Some of these ideas look really great on paper and their flaws only present themselves when applied in the clinic. Happily, most of the really big ideas contained in premodern writings have been distilled into modern TCM already. It is the subtle nuances often contained in this literature which are often glossed over and left out of more streamlined modern text books written for beginners.

Also at issue is exactly what is being said. It is often difficult even for native speaking scholars of Chinese medicine to agree on an interpretation of a given passage in the premodern literature. Premodern Chinese is often terse at best and commentaries on the content of the classics tend to vary widely. One has only to look at the range of commentary on any given chapter of Unschuld's translation of the *Nan Jing* to get a sense of the wide range of possible interpretation. Traditionally, these classics have been percieved much like a fine thread on which the pearls of an oral tradition have been strung. I am not suggesting that this situation should be a deterence to studying the classics. Each of us is capable of making our own decisions over time as to the usefulness of a given work or passage. It has been my experience when researching a specific case, however, that referencing premodern writings tends to be time consuming, and this approach often raises more questions than it answers.

Modern TCM textbooks, on the other hand, contain a synthesis of the most enduring and relevent ideas in the evolution Chinese medicine presented in what is essentially an outline format. Here the chaff has been been winnowed from the wheat. While some of the wheat is inevitably discarded as well, most of what is contained in modern textbooks is clinically useful, if somewhat simplified. Practitioners in the West often complain, however, that their clients do not look like the patterns described in these books. This may reflect a fundamental misunderstanding as to the intent of textbooks in the overall scheme of the Chinese medical literature, and educational process within Chinese medicine in general. The patterns, illnesses, and formulas detailed in textbooks are basically archetypes and were never intended to mirror exactly the idiosyncracies of an individual. Rather, they represent only the basic framework of operation.

This becomes clear when one compares the signs and symptoms for a single pattern presented in several Chinese texts or manuals. Though they often vary in their details, the underlying disease mechanisms at work are understood and all of the varying signs and symptoms are equally possible, most authors will only choose a limited selection of these signs and symptoms in order to convey the type of symptoms one might expect to meet. In other words, textbook descriptions of various patterns are emblematic and not categorically complete in their details.

The experience gained by clinical practice is therefore essential to flesh out these literary bones. In terms of the medical literature, this necessity is reflected in the written record of a practitioner's clinical experience with a specific illness seen in a specific individuals, in other words, in case histories and medical discussions. Case histories by experienced clinicians are a missing link in our entire conception in the West of what the Chinese medical reference literature should look like. While we are just beginning to develop our library of premodern sources and reference textbooks, almost no work has been done in bringing the vast body of case history literature to English speaking practitioners. Translations of case history material by Chen, Wang, and Hsu stand as notable exceptions in the literature.[1],[2]

Perhaps more important than the lack of case histories themselves is the more fundamental lack of appreciation of the role of case histories in the practice and literature of TCM. I would

---

1 *Acupuncture Case Histories From China*, ed. by Chen Ji-rui & Nissi Wang, Eastland Press, Seattle, 1988

2 Otsaku, Keisetsu, *30 Years of Kanpo, Selected Case Studies of an Herbal Doctor*, Oriental Healing Arts Institute, Los Angeles, 1984

argue that, for the reasonably informed professional clinician researching a specific case, case histories are of much greater utility than the premodern classics themselves. The most relevant concepts and ideas pertaining to a given illness and pattern can be readily gleaned from a selection of pertinent case histories. By the very nature of Chinese medical case histories, clinical utility is emphasized over purely theoretical considerations. In researching difficult cases, I will resort to other sources only after a search of my library of case history literature has proven fruitless. To be sure Zhong Zhong-jing's observation in *Prescriptions from the Golden Chamber* that

> ...a person suffering from abdominal fullness and fever for ten days, who has a floating and rapid pulse and eats and drinks as usual should take *Hou Pu Chi Wu Tang*...

is a lucid example of clinical acumen.[3] I doubt, however, if many of us keep such tidbits in our heads, or take the time to directly reference such a quote, even though it has been translated into English. It is far more practical to reference available materials on abdominal fullness where one is likely to see the prescription used, and it is not uncommon to see the above mentioned quote used in the course of Chinese language discussions on abdominal fullness and in pertinent case histories.

There are two branches of the Chinese medical literature directly pertaining to clinical writings. The first is the case history [*yi an*] which is a physician's written record of his or her evaluation, diagnosis, and treatment of a given patient. This genre has a venerable tradition in its own right. The first collection of case

---

3 Chang Chung-Ching, *Prescriptions from the Golden Chamber*, trans. by Wang Su-yen & Hong Yen-hsu, Oriental Healing Arts Institute, 1983, p. 66

histories dates to the Han Dynasty and was written by the famous physician Chun Yu-yi. The second is the medical discussion [*yi huo*]. These include personal ideas on a given medical topic. They have no fixed format and may or may not include case histories.

The fifty volume compendium *Zhong Guo Yi Xue Da Cheng (The Great Compendium of Chinese Medical Theory)* from the Qing dynasty is an anthology of what were considered the most important medical writings throughout Chinese history up to that time. Amongst the volumes ranging from the *Nei Jing* to topics such as pediatrics and otorhinolaryngology are six volumes devoted exclusively to the case histories and medical discussions of various eminent physicians. Medical theses comprise another six volumes in the compendium. This branch of medical writings is clearly well established in the premodern literature. Unschuld's translation of the *Yi Xue Yuan Liu Lun (The Source Flow of Medicine)* is essentially an anthology of medical theses and discussions by its author Hsu Ta-ch'un.

Case histories and medical discussions often blend together. What is recorded as a case history *per se*, may often simply be a platform for a lengthy commentary on the treatment of a given *bian zheng* for a specific illness. Some medical discussions on the other hand turn out to be little more than collections of case histories with a common *bian bing* or *bian zheng*. It is not uncommon for an individual practitioner to identify a very few patterns [*bian zheng*] with a given disease entity [*bian bing*] based on his or her experience in treating that problem. This, of course, is a two edged sword for the reader studying a number of writers

---

4 Unschuld, Paul P., *Forgotten Traditions of Ancient Chinese Medicine, A Chinese View from the Eighteenth Century*, Paradigm Press, Brookline, MA, 1990

on a given topic. There may be times when they are all essentially in agreement as to the best overall conceptual framework for dealing with a given problem and differ only in details, such as the ideal medicinals to be used in prescription modification. Some prescriptions for a given problem will be empirical and universal, such as Xu Xiao-zhou's first prescription for pediatric diarrhea. He advocates its use for any type of pediatric diarrhea. This presents a relatively neat package for the clinician. On the other hand, there may be such a wide range of viewpoints to choose from that the reader is simply overwhelmed. Some authors emphasize detailed diagnostic parameters and subtle modifications of formulas. Contrary views tend to be the rule rather than the exception in Chinese medical literature. It is in the latter case, however, that one is most likely to find a meaningful approach to the treatment of a difficult case.

Having understood the importance of the Chinese case history literature within the context of studying and practicing Chinese medicine, a decision must be made whether premodern cases or contemporary cases are the most useful. It is difficult to become a truly skilled practitioner of Chinese herbal medicine without assimilating at least some of the historical context from which it springs. The great masters of herbal medicine were themselves largely scholars. In this light, it makes sense to read the premodern literature in some depth. During every period in Chinese history, the authors of that time built upon the groundwork laid by their predecessors. Modern writings are the most current expression of this trend, often synthesizing entire strains of thought in a discussion on a given topic. This not only saves the reader the task of going elsewhere to do his or her historical homework but weeds out approaches which have been proven clinically irrelevant. It is often simply more time and energy efficient to concentrate on contemporary sources. In addition, the contemporary trend of incorporating a modern Western disease categorization into the practice of TCM is, I think, a great step forward. While a precise discrimination of patterns (*bian zheng*) should by now be an integral part of any clinicians practice of TCM, the importance of a discrimination of illnesses (*bian bing*) is often neglected. While the forte of TCM is pattern discrimination, Western medicine excels at *bian bing* or disease diagnosis. Such *bian bing* allows for further precision in diagnosis and therapy and I support its incorporation into the TCM methodology. The utility of such an approach is demonstrated in the chapters on gall bladder disease and hypertension. For these reasons I have chosen modern case histories and discussions for this book.

Acupuncture theory forms the foundation for virtually all the permutations of Chinese medicine. The *Nei Jing* and *Nan Jing* predate by 200 years or more the *Shang Han Lun-Jin Gui Yao Lue*, the first works proposing any theoretical framework for the practice of herbal medicine. Nonetheless, TCM theory has developed along predominantly herbal lines. While this TCM methodology has been applied to acupuncture with varying degrees of success, many of the fine points of TCM diagnosis and treatment have been lost in this translation. For instance, the distinction between quickening the blood and actually cracking the blood in the case of masses and tumors has little therapeutic relevance in acupuncture practice where the pertinent points remain largely the same. Yet such a distinction can make the difference between success and failure in herbal medicine. While acupuncture is an important modality in the arsenal of Chinese medicine, it is my feeling that some of its brilliance becomes tarnished when it is placed within the rigid confines of a purely TCM framework.

The limited case history literature on Chinese medicine currently available in English deals largely with acupuncture. Put simply, the herbal case history literature is uncharted territory, and it makes sense to focus some attention on this aspect of Chinese medicine. While herbal in nature, Hsu's translation of Oketsu's case studies represents a distinctly different approach to herbal medicine from the TCM methodology. Since herbal medicine is the hallmark of TCM practice, it is essential to have a representative record of just how it is clinically applied in all its detail. For these reasons the case histories in this volume deal with the practice of herbal medicine only.

Rather than selecting a single case history or discussion from a wide range of topics, I have chosen to present a number of case histories by various authors on a limited number of diseases in the hope that this will provide a more useful base of reference for the topics covered. A single case history may or may not be useful when researching a case, but a collection of case histories on a given topic will almost certainly contain something of value for the clinician. Illnesses were chosen which, I felt, were fairly common in Western practice and yet were poorly represented in the English literature. Internal medicine, gynecology, pediatrics, and *wai ke*[5], the major areas of practice, are represented in this collection. My intent has been to give the reader some sense of the variety inherent in the case history literature. Toward this end, the case histories included here have been translated from the writings of a wide range of authors obtained from a variety of different collections. Also included is the rather new specialty of andrology, or *nan ke*. This refers specifically to disorders of the male urogenital tract. My intent has been to give the reader some sense of the variety inherent in the Chinese case history literature.

Patients in Asia differ from those in the West in a variety of ways and for a variety of reasons. The cultural values and assumptions of one people may engender a very different view of

---

5 *Wai ke* refers to diseases on the external part of the body. The exterior of the body in TCM is defined as the skin, flesh, sinews, and bones.

health and illness from that of another people. The patients I experienced in Chinese clinics were primarily concerned with rather concrete health issues. The issues of personal growth and quality of life which cause my own patients here in the West so much suffering were largely absent in the Chinese patients I saw. They were, for the most part, simply concerned with being able to function in their world. The question may be raised then as to whether Chinese case histories are indeed relevant to Western patients at all. To be sure, a reference library of case histories and medical discussions by eminent TCM physicians in the West would be preferable to looking abroad. However, such an eventuality does not appear to be immediately forthcoming. Furthermore, the patterns described in TCM are fundamental reflections of the human condition as a whole. They may differ in how they are combined from ethnic group to ethnic group or, for that matter, from climatic region to climatic region, but they are universal. As a clinician in the West, one may or may not find a Chinese case history which approximates the case one is researching. However, with even a small selection of Chinese case histories on a specific disease, an understanding will be gained as to the salient issues at play in that disease entity and how those features shape a diagnosis and treatment. Bits and pieces of empirical wisdom will often come forth as well. These frequently have a wide scope of applicability beyond the context of the specific pattern discrimination in which they may appear. Information such as this make Chinese case histories and medical discussions an essential component of the English research literature.

Included in two chapters are some comments of my own. The introduction to the chapter on gallbladder disease and the case histories in that chapter were originally published in a somewhat modified format in the *Journal of the College of Traditional Chinese Medicine* and include my views on the utility of a Western discrimination of illnesses. While compiling the chapter on pediatric diarrhea, it occurred to me that many practitioners shy away from this area of endeavor because of problems in compliance in actually administering Chinese herbs to children in the West. I have, therefore, included some of my own ideas on this matter. While these are germane to the issue of pediatric practice in general, they do not pertain specifically to pediatric diarrhea.

Introducing this collection of writings is an essay by Qin Bo-wei. One of the foremost doctors of TCM of the 20th Century, Qin was a prolific writer and researcher of the classical medicla literature as well as a renowned clinician. The depth of his understanding of the *Nei Jin* and *Nan Jing* was so well known that in Shanghai he was referred to as Qin Nei Jing. Qin's 1958 essay on case histories is one of the most articulate statements addressing the place of case histories in the Chinese medical literature of this century. His fondness for the case histories of the physicians of the Qing Dynasty is evident in his many references to them throughout the essay. In 1939 Qin Bo-wei edited an anthology of the best case writings of the Qing Dynasty, titled *Qing Dai Ming Yi Yi Huo Jing Hua (The Essential Medical Discourses of the Famous Physicians of the Qing Dynasty)*, and this earlier work clearly provides a reference base for his discussion of case histories. Qin's essay on the relevance of case studies to clinical practice has been translated here in its entirety as an inspiration to readers in the West.

How to use case histories

While I believe that reading and researching the case histories of eminent physicians is central to deepening one's practice of Chinese medicine, case histories will not do your thinking for you. A formula can rarely be lifted directly from a case history and used unmodified elsewhere. The value of case histories is that they provide a truer picture of real life patients. Because the signs and symptoms of one's own patients will typically vary, at least somewhat, from the signs and symptoms presented in the case, the protocols in that case will usually have to be modified to more perfectly fit one's patient. Based on my own fumblings with Chinese case histories, I would like to suggest some practical ideas for their use.

1. Do a complete diagnosis of your own first, including both disease and pattern discriminations. If the patient does not already have a Western disease diagnosis, the TCM practitioner should include a traditional Chinese diagnosis *e.g.*, *wei tong*, stomach pain, *lin zheng*, stranguria, or *xiao ke*, thirsting and wasting. Write everthing down — pulse, tongue, signs, and symptoms — using standard professional terminology and especially a clear, concise pattern discrimination diagnosis. We sometimes make assumptions in our heads that are clearly questionable when rendered on paper. You will be comparing your own findings in a given case with those of someone who is hopefully more experienced than yourself in treating the problem at hand. While practitioners vary in the amount of information they provide in case histories, it's best not to start with insufficient data on your end.

You may find that a practitioner is big on a diagnostic parameter which you had not investigated. For instance, some doctors find that the color and quality of the nasal cavity itself is an important consideration in treating deep source nasal congestion. Go back and check it out. Many modern physicians in the People's Republic of China make use of Western diagnostic tests such as urinalysis, gastroscopy, and ultrasound. If your patient has been evaluated in this way, its nice to have access to these even if they are not immediately meaningful to you. They may become relevant in light of the cases you are referencing and you may learn something along the way.

2. If your diagnosis is similar to none of the patterns in the discussions you have available, then re-evaluate it. Do not necessarily revise it. If all your sources say that there should be a component of liver counterflow and you do not see this, then it may not be there. But at least you have specifically looked for it. Make a note to yourself in the patient's chart to be on the lookout for these common patterns which do not quite fit your case. You may see hints of it cropping up as treatment progresses.

3. Remember, you are not trying to fit your case into someone's elses case history or discussion anymore than you are trying to lock your case into a single rigid pattern. Find the patterns and the case histories that are relevant to the case. It may be that none of the discussions that are available to you speak to your case at all. That is okay. It's better to not use that material than to force a fit. You can be sure that the nifty but presently unusable idea you have uncovered will stick in your mind the next time a similar situation comes up and you may get to use it then. Nothing is wasted.

4. In actuality it's somewhat rare to get a perfect fit. Often I find myself snatching relevant bits of information from a number of different cases when trying to cobble together a diagnosis, treatment plan, and prescription. While I said above that you should have a diagnosis in hand before you start reading case histories, you may find that precision in someone else's thinking on a given problem helps you to hone yours both diagnostically and therapeutically. Its okay to go back and search for components you have overlooked, but, if you have a solid diagnostic framework to move around in, the whole thing is less likely to disintegrate into a ball of confusion before your eyes.

5. Most cases you read have progressed in a reasonably smooth manner. Yours may not. With few exceptions, people put only

their most sterling work on display in writing. This is unfortunate because understanding an error is every bit as useful as beholding a triumph. Studying how cases progress in general can give you a sense of whether or not you are on track with your treatment plan. However, do not assume that your patient will necessarily progress in as tidy a manner as the patients in Chinese case histories.

One of the most reassuring things for to me to read in any case history is that the patient returns improved but with some complication, like diarrhea or insomnia, that has to be modified for. The writer will not often state that this is a result of some miscalculation on his part but will simply note that the greasy, Radix Coquitus Rehmanniae was removed and substituted with Rhizoma Polygonati or that Cortex Albizziae and Radix Polygalae were added to the prescription to calm the spirit. The realities of clinical practice come through, nevertheless, if one reads between the lines, and we see that even master physicians may craft a prescription which is initially too greasy, agitating, or otherwise imperfect. Sometimes practitioners will note that the treatment measures of supplementing the spleen and transforming dampness in the case of longstanding diarrhea were not enough and additional measures for astringing the intestines were required. I personally have found this sort of reporting quite empowering. While we all try to do our best to get it right on the first shot, it's somehow comforting to know that even senior practitioners may need a few passes to sort things out.

6. In researching a number of different cases which have the same *bian bing* and similar *bian zheng*, you may find a discussion or even a specific case which is particularly relevant to the cases you see. Because of their utility in your pratice, its worth memorizing them or at least keeping them at hand if they are not prescriptions with which you are already familiar. I am slowly developing a repertory of favorite cases which speak most

directly to the kinds of patterns I tend to see for a given illness. This will vary geographically as well as from clinician to clinician. I keep my eye out, for instance, for case histories and discussions involving hot asthmas with dry phlegm since I see alot more of these in Colorado than the runny, wet, cold asthmas more common in damp, cold climates.

Concluding remarks

It is my feeling that the development of a body of Chinese medical case histories in the English language is the single most important aspect of the Chinese medical literature to which Western readers currently require access. That is not to say that more basic texts and clinical manuals are unnecessary, nor have all the medical classics been adequately translated. However, for graduate practitioners in clinical practice, case histories are the most valuable source of useful information on the treatment of real-life patients. This is particularly true in light of the the fact that many acupuncture schools are able to provide clinical experience which is limited at best and which is often not supervised by truly seasoned practitioners.[6]

Having acknowledged the relevance of the clinically oriented Chinese medical literature to the Western practice of Chinese medicine, the question inevitably arises as to how clinicians will

---

6 When I was in acupuncture school, two of my most influential teachers there, Kiiko Matsumoto and Steven Birch, published their first book, ***Five Elements & Ten Stems***. It contained a number of case histories by eminent Japanese acupuncturists. I remember asking Kiiko why she hadn't included any cases of her own. She looked at me as if I had asked her to perform brain surgery and replied that she felt that she was not experienced enought to have anything clinically useful to offer. This was at a time when she was among the most experienced clinicians at the school.

access this literature. At this point, a call for more extensive translation of the case history literature, while admirable, is not likely to be very fruitful. There are currently very few people translating Chinese medicine into English, and the task of translating more substantial works is simply more compelling, both from an academic and economic standpoint. Given time, Western practitioners of TCM are themselves more likely to produce an English language case history literature. Unfortunately, senior physicians in the West who are willing to take the time to publish their insights are as scarce as translators of Chinese medicine seem to be. The obvious solution to this conundrum is for practitioners of TCM in general to learn to read Chinese. I am not suggesting that it is necessary for our acpuncture schools to produce practitioner-sinologists. I do believe, however, that a basic understanding of the mother language of Chinese medicine is a fundamental necessity for the further development of our profession.

Over the course of my studies in acupuncture school, I had the good fortune to learn a rudimentary level of medical Chinese. More than any of the other classes I attended, this provided me with the tools necessary to proceed along the path of Chinese medicine. Learning the Chinese language can be a daunting prospect. While under his tutelage, one of my Chinese instructors celebrated his 20th year of being baffled by Chinese. It seemed that there was always some aspect of his area of specialty, Chinese Buddhist studies, which eluded him. On the other hand, once I learned even a few hundred characters and some basic grammar, I was amazed at the doors which opened to me. It seemed that a vast amount of information was immediately at my fingertips. I remember our teacher balking at our requests that we translate case histories in class. He felt that the grammar and vocabulary in them was too simple and would teach us little. Many of his students, on the other hand, saw the incredible clinical potential in these simple case histories and would have been content to linger for a while in these seemingly shallow waters. Instead, we pushed on into the depths of the *Qian Jin Yao Fang* and *Su Wen* and tore our hair out.

The fact is that an advanced degree in sinological studies is not required in order to gain clinical access to most modern case histories and medical discussions. The needs of the clinician are not necessarily those of the scholar, and a rudimentary understanding of how the Chinese language is written can provide access to hundreds of times more literature than is currently or ever likely to be available in English. At this level, although useful, it is not even essential to be able to speak Chinese at all. Given some basic general vocabulary, one's character recognition may be largely confined to Chinese medical terminology. The vocabulary used in modern Chinese medical writing is actually quite limited, and skill in the use of a Chinese-English dictionary fills in the inevitable gaps in one's reading comprehension. Simply being able to read the symptoms, diagnosis, and acupuncture or herbal prescription in a case history can have immense therapeutic potential even if some of the fine points are lost. Even a rudimentary knowledge of Chinese among the ranks of Western practitioners of TCM would have the potential to significantly raise the level of discussion and translation in our profession. The gap between the "experts" who will brook no challenge from the uninitiated and the TCM working stiff who must take the word of the pundits on every matter would begin to narrow. At the very least, the questions by practitioners posed to their Chinese and Western teachers and their peers will potentially be more considered and articulate.

To be sure, medical Chinese at the entry level has its limitations. Much, if not most of the premodern Chinese medical literature is likely to remain tantalizingly out of reach. Access to premodern Chinese requires a much greater investment of time and effort and demands another level of competence altogether.

Although they are inexorably intertwined, at some point one has to decide whether one is going to be primarily a sinologist or a clinician. Even the training of TCM physicians in the People's Republic of China does not necessarily include classical Chinese. Virtually all of the Chinese medical classics, however, have renderings in modern Chinese, complete with annotations and modern commentaries. While these are a step removed from the originals, these modern versions serve as an accessible bridge for the persevering student.

In summary, if one makes the initial effort to learn Chinese at the "entry level" outlined above, he or she will have acccss to more clinically based information than they can ever read in a lifetime. The case histories and medical discussions collected in this volume require a relatively low level of competence in reading the Chinese language to access. They are presented here as an example of what is readily available to anyone with such an entry level ability. Over the years, the encouragement and enthusiasm my mentors have given me in pursuing my translational efforts has been tremendously empowering and perhaps some of that excitement and inspiration will infect others. It is my hope that this anthology is a step, however faltering, in that direction.

ON WRITING A CHINESE MEDICAL CASE HISTORY

by Qin Bo-wei

From the numerous clinical summary reports published in Chinese medical journals in recent years, it is not difficult to see that the therapies of these Chinese doctors are effective. All this [publishing] has laid a foundation for the arrangement and enhancement [of information in these fields]. For statistical convenience, these summary reports are generally composed along Western medical models including gender, age, symptomology, laboratory tests, general treatment, and rate of recovery. Of course this is all very good and exceedingly necessary. Still, as an exchange of experience, in a certain percentage of [these reports,] the use of this format fails to illustrate the content of the treatment. Most practitioners feel that [the format of these reports] is difficult to follow and to popularize. Also, such reports very seldom contain detailed explanations of Chinese medical pattern discriminations.[1] Old Chinese doctors are not adept at this sort of reporting. Although they do support the collection of these valuable bits of experience lest they be lost, they nonetheless feel that few cases can be done in this inconvenient style. As a result of this, I believe that aside from summary reports, a need remains for a resurgance of [more traditional] Chinese medical customs [in case reporting]. On the one hand, these should seek to conform to the demands of the present styles while, on the other, assimilating extensive clinical experi-

---

1 This has changed considerably since 1958 when this article was written

ence. Medical cases specific to Chinese medicine are practical, realistic, vivid, and vigorous, and it is most appropriate that Chinese doctors work together reviewing and learning from each other's work. It is essential that extenive anthologies of this material be published in a timely manner.

In the past, whenever a Chinese doctor wrote out a prescription, there was a pulse record, an accounting of symptomology, etiology, diagnosis, and treatment. In utilizing such prescriptions, later practitioners retained this format in their selections for publication and these are, therefore, referred to as case histories, or *yi an*. Examples such as Ye Tian-shi's *Lin Zheng Zhi Nan* (*The Guidebook of Clinical Symptomology*) are a representative record of the prescriptions of the day. This is also referred to as the *Ye Tian-shi Yi-An (Case Histories of Ye Tian-shi).* The initial prescriptions and subsequent modifications written for a single disease may be presented in a notetaking [essay] format. These are essentially a combination of the [style described] above and the traditional case history or *yi an*. In order to conveniently differentiate them, [the former] are at times referred to as medical discussions or *yi huo*. Regardless of whether it is a case history or a medical discussion, all [case records] are based upon clinical facts which are then summarized with a theory, followed by measures [for treatment]. These theories and principles all have a definitive basis [in the medical literature]. Some case histories offer practical [*i.e.*, clinical] confirmation of the classical literature, and some offer quotes from the various schools, [thus generating] ongoing and lively discussion which is without the slightest restraint. In this way, even if conditions are encountered which cannot be found in the literature, they too can be dealt with in an ingenious and rational manner.

Therefore, the characteristics of a [useful] medical case are as follows: 1) They possess a guiding and enlightening quality, offering an ample reflection of the spirit of independent thinking and skillful utilization [of prescriptions and medicinals]. 2) They leave no leeway for variant mechanisms, holding to a single illness and a single [appropriate] prescription or medicine. This is as opposed to the scrambling of prescriptions which have been simply thrown together devoid of any organization.

Once a beginning student of Chinese medicine is capable of comprehending basic theory and the rules of treatment, he can simultaneously integrate clinical [experience] and refer to case histories. How else can one understand how theory is employed to differentiate patterns, how theory is confirmed by means of practice, and how a standard prescription is appropriately modified? [One must] learn where to use common techniques in the odd emergency situation and grasp the relationships of the positions advocated by each school when they arise. Even for private practitioners, case histories are regarded as a borrowed lens, offering an opportunity to learn from the strong points of others, increase one's wisdom, and continuously enhance the level of their profession. The following quote illustrates this point.

In the case histories of Xue Sheng-bai, he quotes the *Jin Gui* [*Yao Lue*] as follows,

> In the case of a male, a large pulse means taxation and an extremely vacuous pulse also means taxation. It is important to understand that a large pulse means taxation resulting from vexation exhaustion injuring the qi, while a vacuous pulse means taxation resulting from lust producing loss [of essence].

The case histories of Wang Xu-gao [state],

> The lungs govern the qi of the body. It is also said that when water exits from the high source, the ancient peoples opened the ghost door to cleanse the viscera.

(The author notes that both these sentences are from the *Nei Jing*, and the inference is that of the promotion of diaphoreses and urination). Although it is said that [diaphoresis and urination] are initiated from *tai yang*, this is actually quite close to the [function of] the lung.

The case histories of Ye Tian-shi [note],

> The *Nei Jing* [says] if there is taxation, then warm it, and when taxation shakes the body, the yang qi is the first to be injured. The meaning of this warm [*wen*] character is to warm and nourish, and it means that one is not warming the competing heat. Injury due to taxation of a longstanding nature is detrimental, and the *Nei Jing* contains a passage [which says, in the case of] detriment, benefit it. To benefit is to fortify *and* benefit. All medicinals which supplement the qi are warm and have a sweet taste. They initially shore up and engender the yang, and this is the main treatment for taxation detriment.

These classical records can be explained by means of clinical observation. Using these classical citations as a guide, a deeper understanding can be gained in the implementation of treatment.

The case histories of Wang Xu-gao [note],

> The *Nei Jing* states that if needles and flints are inapplicable, then use sweet tasting medicines.

The *Jin Gui* concurs, advising the use of ***Huang Qi Jian Zhong Tang*** in order to increase the appetite and promote an effulgence of fluids.

The medical records of Ye Tian-shi [note],

> Zhang Zhong-jing states that diaphoresis may not be induced where there are warm pathogens. As diaphoresis

plunders fluids and injures yin, the body will certainly become scorched. If this is repeated, one's life will be shortened. It also says that with snoring and difficult speech, severe cases of fright palpitations, twitching, and convulsions, this is due to nothing more than a drastic plundering of fluids. In modern illnesses with fever, the pattern tends not to be that of a pathogenic visitation within the *tai yang*, and it is a mistake to throw in *Qiang* [*Huo*, Rhizoma Notopterygii] and *Fang* [*Feng*, Radix Ledebouriellae] which are spicy, warm, and induce diaphoresis.

Of course there is the common possibility that the upper orifices are not assimilating and the lower orifices are not eliminating. Therefore, extreme purgation to drain heat might be employed, yet the force with which this plunders fluids and injures yang is rarely appreciated. Such rash purgation will plunder fluids and, moreover, cause yin to perish. In observing the discussions of Zhong-jing where the pathogen is slight and the vacuity great, if the yin humors and yang fluids have dried up as well, *Fu Mai Tang* should be administered, as this reflects his original intent.

The interrelationships between the various source texts are evident in these quotes. This [example] illustrates the fact that Zhong-jing's medical principles were based on his understanding and experience of the *Nei Jing*, and some of [Zhong-jing's] greatest developments came in the treatment of warm disease. Ye Tian-shi was the leading proponent of the school of warm disease, his theoretical extrapolations being related directly to the *Shang Han Lun*. While there are those who arbitrarily separate [the school of warm disease from] the *Nei Jing*, *Shang Han Lun*, and *Jin Gui*, emphasizing the opposition of injury by cold and warm illness, this clearly·a myopic point of view.

To further [illustrate this point] the medical records of Wang Xu-gao note,

In former days, the pathomechanism of clouding mania[2] lay in the *yang ming*, and so methods of forceful purgation were used. Today, with abdominal distension, a white tongue, and fine pulse, the pathomechanism lies within the *tai yang*, and so it is important to [employ] spicy, warm medicines to penetrate the yang and transport movement of the middle pivot. Flexibility based on changes in the [patho]mechanism, and [treatment] of the acute [manifestation] should be primary. No comment should be made as to the superiority of [therapeutic models based on] cold or heat.

The medical records of Wu Ju-tong [note],

Zhong-jing said that *tai yang* [illness] arrives in five or six days, and if these *tai yang* symptoms are not alleviated, then the *tai yang* should be expelled and *Gui Zhi Tang* is indicated. If there is slight pain in the head and body, with a consequent fever and no aversion to wind cold, this indicates that *tai yang* has not been alleviated and *Gui Zhi Tang* is logically indicated. However, if this patient is suffering from damp heat, does not like sweets, and has a slight cough, the deletion of the sweet medicines and inclusion of spicy, dry medicinals is necessary in the administration of *Gui Zhi Tang*.

The medical records of Ye Tian-shi note:

The opinion of times past was that *Si Jun Zi Tang* nourished the spleen/stomach and promoted harmonious flow. Incorporation of Folium Mori Albi (*Sang Ye*) and Cortex Radicis Moutan (*Dan Pi*) [into this prescription, so as to] treat fire in the wood of *shao yang* and to lessen the errosion to the earth, is, in this case, spurious. Suppose that

---

2 This refers to clouding of the sensorium, especially the vision, with mania.

> within the body there was an illness due to disharmony caused by an affront to the two qi[3], and the pulse indicates extreme damage. How could such [withered] grass and wood ever regain vitality? In observing and treating this disease it is of no benefit to boost the qi with the imprecise applications of medicinals, and this should not be the basis of treatment. In the case of diminished appetite and diarrhea, it is inappropriate to administer greasy, enriching [medicines]. Therefore, the temporary use of measures such as Jing-yue's *Li Yin Qian,* combined with the principles of calming counterflow, securing and containing, [the leakage of qi are indicated in order to treat this condition].

These [examples] further illustrate that our predecessors used medicines according to the symptoms, making constitutional considerations and precisely modifying standard prescritions. If treatment was not successful, they would speak out without reservation, and this attitude is of particular value.

Many peculiarities of treatment are recorded within case histories. An example of this is Wang Xu-gao's treatment of pediatric emaciation with symptoms of jaundice, copious phlegm, anorexia, a slight daytime cough, and a sound in the throat while sleeping at night. Because children are inherently adverse to taking medicines, the medicinal date technique was used. Take Radix Panacis Ginseng (*Ren Shen*), Rhizoma Atractylodis Macrocephalae (*Bai Zhu*), Sclerotium Poriae Cocoris (*Fu Ling*), Cortex Magnoliae Officinalis (*Hou Po*), Semen Torreyae (*Fei Zi*), Radix Praeparatus Glycyrrhizae (*Zhi Gan Cao*), Pericarpium Citri Reticulatae (*Chen Pi*), Bulbus Fritillariae Thunbergii (*Bei Mu*), treated Rhizoma Pinelliae Ternatae (*Zhi Ban Xia*), Tuber Ophiopogonis Japonicae (*Mai Dong*), and Rhizoma Atractylodis (*Cang Zhu*) and grind into a fine powder. Remove the seeds from the dates and put 2 *fen* of this powder into each date. Bind

---

3 The two qi here refer to yin and yang.

well with thread. Semen Tinglizi (*Ting Li*) may be used also, with the dates being cooked in water to warm and soften them, afterwards dry in the sun. One piece should be chewed carefully when the child is hungry, and 5-6 may be taken daily.

Another example [of the unique insights which have been recorded in case literature] is Zhang Jin-qing's treatment of intense cough due to injury by wind. [In this case], an affliction by cold is contracted following recovery [from an earlier illness]. ***San Ao Tang*** is used, but there is concern due to its bitter, warm, coursing, and dispersing nature. Therefore, therapy is a modified version of lung distillation [*fei lu*]. [In this version of the treatment,] water is not dripped on the pig's lung, the nodes of Herba Ephedrae Sinensis (*Ma Huang*), the skin and tips of Semen Pruni Armeniacae (*Xing Ren*), and the nodes of Radix Glycyrrhizae (*Gan Cao*) are not discarded, and this steamed distillate is administered warm.

In addition, there are a number of simple prescriptions and empirical prescriptions with coordinated preparation [methods]. Ye Tian-shi's treatment of obstructed menstruation causing concommitant suppuration from the ear is an example. In the pulse report[4] it indicates,

> When the [patient is] recumbent administer one *qian* of ***Cha Tiao San***. Pare the tip off a piece of Radix Euphorbiae Kansui (*Gan Sui*), insert it into the patients's ear, and hold

---

4 In a pulse report (*mai an*), the writer gives specific information regarding the treatment of a specific condition, but is not referring to a specific individual whom he or she has treated. For instance, in the Qing dynasty discussion of patterns *Lei Zheng Zhi Zai* by Lin Pei, every illness discussed is followed by a series of *mai an* by other well known physicians. A pulse report may also simply reflect the physician's pulse finding in a given case. Qin Bo-wei uses the term in this context later in the essay.

> a small one half *cun* piece of Radix Glycyrrhizae (*Gan Cao*) in the mouth.

In Xue Sheng-bai's treatment of wheezing cough, aside from using prescriptions for boosting the qi and supplementing the lung, he also indicated in his pulse cases,

> In the morning or evening catch one otter [*lai*] and dry its liver in the shade. Grind Colla Cornu Cervi (*Lu Jiao Jiao*) on the end of a wooden pestle in a mortar. Administer 1 *qian* of the Colla Cornu Cervi in the morning and administer 1 *qian* of the otter liver in the evening. Both are to be taken with boiled water. This is a commonly used technique.

In summary, case histories are a [unique] expression of the synthesis of theory and practice. [Please] bear with these abundant examples and the fact that the passages extracted are from the Qing Dynasty only. The entire leopard may be inferred [from each of the spots in its coat]. Case histories reflect the success of a given physician in treating illness, and each phycian's attempts to treat an illness should inevitably be recorded in case histories. Our predecessors have retained and passed on [this information]. In the wake of these historical developments, today's physicians should have many outstanding specific collections and arrangements of these case histories.

While it is understood that the authors of books on case histories must be high level [practitioners], there are sometimes unnecessary misgivings [as to whether one is qualified to record one's cases]. The case histories of our predecesors were, for the most part, [written] in the popular style and language of the time and with the intent that even the patient might understand them.[5] For instance, the case histories of Yu Zai-jin note,

> When the face, eyes, and body become entirely jaundiced, there is no glomus oppression and urination is normal, this was referred to by Zhong-jing as vacuity jaundice, and so [Zhang Zhong-jing's] treatment techniques should be used.

Case histories of Wang Jiu-feng offer [the following insights],

> Once medication has been administered pain should not occur. If indeed pain does not occur then [the patient is cured]. If pain does develop, the patient will find it unbearable; however, once it ceases the patient will instantly feel well.

> In the case of rapid movement within the five phases, nothing can surpass wind and fire. Depressive fire and depressive wind as well as stasis of qi and dampness may engender parasites. If the parasites are not exterminated, then the wind cannot be dispersed and fire cannot be cooled. [In this case] depression cannot be supplemented, nor can it be cracked.

> In regulating the *chong* and *ren*, disinhibiting the *yang ming*, and melding and harmonizing the qi and blood, although the menses is [not directly] treated, is regulated of its own accord.

These arrangements of symptoms and theoretical discussions are explained so clearly that even an old woman could understand them and they are all [written] without a trace of pretension. Another example may be found in the case histories of Zhang

---

5 Qin Bo-wei's point is that one need not be a scholar or master physician to have something useful to contribute to the case literature.

Jin-qing which contain milk, bread, and Western medicinals. The case histories of Jin Zi-jiu contain protein, and those of Ding Gan-ren employ new terminology in recording the treatment of pneumonia and body temperature.[6] It must be understood that the methodology of writing case histories is not the same as that of an essay, and its sole strong point is that it is an honest and straightforward report.

Naturally, we ought to point out that as civilization developed, the language of the ancients evolved as well. Thus, the methodology for composing case histories in modern times should also be discussed. In more recent times, the words and sentences have been simplified and crucial issues have been thoroughly discussed. Toward a better arrangement of case histories, I have drafted six criteria for consideration.

1. Regardless of whether the condition is common, difficult, or miscellaneous, it should be collected if it is potentially useful for clinical reference. Of course there must be some elucidation [on the case], and there should generally be more on the treatment of commonly seen illnesses. This should inspire us to strive for more and better measures in the treatment of commonly seen illnesses. If we ignore these commonly seen illnesses in favor of difficult and mixed illnesses, the efficacy of Chinese medicine will be diminished.

2. [Case reporting should] not be limited to cases in which the illness was cured, but include cases where the treatment was not effective, where treatment was first erroneous and then corrected, or was erroneous and then fatal. All need to be collected equally. Failure provides experience so that others may avoid

---

6 Qin Bo-wei illustrates here that even modern insights may be rendered within the traditional format of case reporting.

travelling down the same disastrous path. It also provides the reference material for further research.

3. When diagnosing illness, one should not be too detailed with pulse histories, nor should one's rhetorical skills be overused, as frank and honest notetaking is of primary importance. When the time arrives to compile pulse cases, they can then be polished. Although excessive alterations are inappropriate, all the information need not be included as long as the distinguishing characteristics of primary importance are selected and especially the turning point in the course of therapy. In order to supplement and clarify [the report], one may also add "remarks".

4. If one uses a notetaking literary style, it is of primary importance that one be frank, honest, concise, and employ common language. It is important not to digress too far from the topic at hand in one's discussions, nor are literary citations necessary.[7]

5. The name of the patient must not be revealed and the name of some [fictitious] comrade may be used as a substitute. Nonetheless, the gender and age must be recorded. The place of birth, occupation, etiology, and progression of the illness should be noted, as well as constitution, season, habits, and customs, and these all must be integrated with the [description of the] illness.

6. The Chinese medical designation of the illness should be indicated in each case history, and while the Western medical diagnosis may be included, the Chinese medical designation is of primary importance. If there is no Chinese name for a given illness, then a Western medical name can certainly be used. However, treatment will nonetheless be based on Chinese

---

7 It is a common practice, however, for physicians to justify a given treatment plan with a citation from the classics.

medical theory, and must be elucidated in "remarks". This is an important issue.

Finally, it should be pointed out that [although] the format of Chinese medical case histories is ancient, their content has undergone an uninterrupted progression. Because they are valued for both their practical applications as well as research, they still merit serious attention in the present day. It is a pity that lately the [use of] pulse reports have been gradually diminishing in Chinese medical precriptions. [Pulse reports] have become all too sketchy, and some hospital workers have abandoned pulse records altogether.

There are those who say that only the names of the medicines should appear on an herbal prescription. [However, if this is done, then] not only does the patient fail to understand which illness is the cause of his suffering, but the physician himself becomes ignorant over a period of time. If this patient seeks diagnosis and treatment from another physician, there is no way to explain the progression of the illness, or what, in reality, is the actual situation. In the springtime I visited Jiangsu Provincial Chinese Medical Hospital. The head of the hospital, Zou Yun-xiang, informed me that he also had a similar feeling [regarding case reporting]. Therefore, in that hospital, except for the regular case history files, pulse records have been reintroduced, and, although these procedures are inevitably troublesome, over the long run this will become a habit. As a result of this, I would include a recommendation that, in the future, when Chinese physicians compose prescriptions, the inclusion of a pulse record should be required. This will not only arrange the pulse records when convenient, but have a definite benefit for both the physician and patient as well. To detractors and proponents alike, I hope you will comment on this!

(1958)

BETWEEN A ROCK AND A HARD PLACE

Discussions of Cholecystitis

Introduction

The yang organs are often given a secondary role by practitioners of Traditional Chinese Medicine (TCM). With the exception of disorders which primarily involve the channels and collaterals, they are, for all practical purposes, largely ignored in the conceptual framework of herbal medicine. Urinary bladder problems are subsumed under the broader categories of kidney and liver disorders while intestinal dysfunctions are most often subsumed under spleen function. The stomach is perhaps the most autonomous of the bowels, and even it is treated largely as a lieutenant of the spleen. Finally there is the gallbladder, which is scarcely spoken of without reference to the liver.

Acupuncturists who are trained in non-TCM traditions often give more equal attention to the yang *fu,* and clearly their usefulness is not as limited as TCM textbooks might make it seem. A closer look at the gallbladder will serve as a good example. The gallbladder stores and secretes bile.[1] It is a shunt of the main biliary pathway which stores and secretes the bile excreted by the liver. When food enters the duodenum, the gallbladder contracts and aids digestion by increasing the emulsifying power of the

---

1 Kaptchuk, Ted, *The Web That Has No Weaver*, Congdon & Weed Inc., New York, 1983, p. 66

pancreatic fluid.[2] Yves Requena has made great strides in reconciling a Western medical understanding of gallbladder function with the Chinese medical understanding. He explains:

> Bile thus aids in the absorption of cholesterol, fatty acids and also liposoluble vitamins (A, D, E, K).[3]
>
> Vitamin A goes into the composition of the visual purple of the retina cells and enables us to see shapes. Its deficiency leads to the loss of night vision.[4]

This, of course, echoes the longstanding association of visual disturbances and liver/gallbladder disorders in Chinese medicine.

> Vitamin D promotes the absorption of calcium and phosphorous in the intestine as it does their fixation in the bones.[5]

And, in Chapter 10 of the *Ling Shu*, we read that

> ...*zu shao yang* (the gallbladder meridian) is involved in all bone disorders,

explaining the placement of the meeting point of the marrow on the gallbladder channel at *Xuanzhong* (GB-39).

---

2 Requena, Yves, M.D., *Terrains And Pathology In Acupuncture*, Paradigm Publications, Brookline, MA, 1986, p. 133

3 Ibid., p. 134

4 Ibid., p. 172

5 Ibid., p. 134

> Vitamin K (phytonadine, menaquine and menadione) is important in the formation of prothrombin by the liver.[6]

With this reference, Requena infers that the gallbladder, by virtue of its absorptive function, assists the liver in producing blood. More classically, the gallbladder is considered one of the so-called curious organs and as such is associated with essence qi. Requena supports this latter association by reminding us that

> Cholesterol is also at the origin of the production of sexual and corticoadrenal steroid hormones.[7]

Ted Kaptchuk, apparently speaking for the modern TCM position, states that,

> These curious organs are actually of little importance in both theory and practice.[8]

This position is short-sighted. The curious organs, including the gallbladder, have the unique quality of resembling the

> Yang organs in form and the Yin organs in function...they store and do not dispense.[9]

When one considers that the liver often behaves like a yang organ, manifesting as hot and replete, it is small wonder that the gallbladder suffers an identity crisis and manifests its pathologic

---

6 Ibid., p. 134

7 Ibid., p. 135

8 Kaptchuk, Ted, op.cit., p. 336

9 Ibid., p. 336

emotion as timidity. The gallbladder distinguishes itself among its brotherly bowels as being the only one that contains a pure substance, *i.e.*, bile, and thus, alone, is considered a pure bowel. A further distinguishing trait is its role as the "judge who decides"[10] leaving the details of strategy to the liver.

Gallbladder pathology is clearly described in the classical literature. The *Ling Shu* states,

> A patient who displays symptoms of frequent vomiting, spitting up of bile, sighing anguish (as if someone wanted to catch them and put them in prison) has a diseased gallbladder. The stomach is also affected as if there were a leak in the bile secretion; this is why the patient's mouth is always bitter.[11]
>
> Obstructions to the throat that create a frequent desire to spit out...[12]

also relate to gallbladder disease.

Disorders of the gallbladder are by no means uncommon. Cecil and Loeb's *Textbook of Medicine*[13] cites cholelithiasis or gallstones as the basic source of gallbladder pathology from the Western medical perspective. Most common diseases are a result

---

10 Requena, Yves, op.cit., p. 136

11 Ibid., p. 143

12 Ibid., p. 144

13 Cecil and Loeb, *Textbook of Medicine*, W.B. Saunders & Co., Philadelphia, 1985

of the presence of stones.[14] Chronic cholecystitis is the most common non-acute manifestation of cholelithiasis. This produces a steady pain in the upper right quadrant or epigastrium, the onset of which may take only a few minutes. It will quickly reach a plateau of intensity that may range from moderate to excruciating and which will gradually decrease over a period of as little as 30 minutes or as much as a few hours. Many patients experience simultaneous pain referred to the back near the scapula or right shoulder. Nausea and vomiting may accompany an attack and some attacks may be related to ingestion of a fatty meal. Episodes may occur daily or as rarely as every few years. Real-time ultrasonography is perhaps the most reliable method of detecting gallstones, as well as the most comprehensive. While dietary changes, anti-cholinergics, and antacids may provide temporary symptomatic relief, cholecystectomy remains the treatment of choice.[15]

Acute cholecystitis will usually produce right subcostal pain and tenderness. However, acute inflammation of the gallbladder is apparent in less than 20 percent of cases diagnosed as acute cholecystitis. Pathological findings of the gallbladder wall and clinical manifestations of gallstone disease correlate poorly as well. This would suggest that the actual source of imbalance from a modern Western medical perspective is as yet undetermined and would admit the possibility that the disharmony might be fundamentally energetic in nature.

Acute cholecystitis usually begins with abdominal pain that increases gradually in severity and is again located in the right subcostal region, but may begin in the upper left quadrant or

---

14 Ibid., p. 853

15 Ibid., p. 857

epigastrium and move as the inflammation progresses. Referred back and shoulder pain is common as well. Murphy's sign may be present, which is described as heightened tenderness in the subhepatic region which arrests inspiration upon palpation. A distended gallbladder may be felt distinctly and is confirmational of a suspected diagnosis in one-third of patients. In the rest it will be unpalpable due to obesity, rigidity of the abdominal wall, a deep subhepatic location, or because it has shrunk due to previous inflammation. Jaundice may be present, caused by edema of the common duct or the presence of calculi in the common duct. Ultrasonography again is the most reliable method of detecting causative stones and surgery is the therapy of choice.[16]

Cholangitis or inflammation of the bile ducts due to calculi obstructing the ducts is considered a potentially serious disease that generally warrants immediate diagnosis and treatment in a hospital setting. Intermittent cholangitis consisting of biliary colic, jaundice, and fever and chills, known as Charcot's triad, is the most common symptom complex. Whether the above symptoms fluctuate together over a span of a few days or weeks, cholangitis from biliary obstruction is the cause. In a typical attack, chills may precede the other symptoms. Epigastric or right upper quadrant pain indistinguishable from gallstone pain is steady and severe. Pain may be referred to the right interscapular area, the upper back, right shoulder, or even the precordia, suggesting coronary artery or esophageal disease. Surgery is the treatment of choice.[17]

---

16 Ibid., p. 857-859

17 Ibid., p. 853

Various medications exist which will dissolve some kinds of stones, including chenodeoxycholate and ursodeoxycholate; however, their effectiveness is partial at best. When treatment is discontinued after initial dissolution, gallstones return in up to 50% of patients within five years. This, of course, reflects the shortsightedness of treating the stones as the fundamental issue rather than as a manifestation of a physio-energetic imbalance.

Clearly the clinical predominance of the liver in the herbal treatment of hepato-biliary disorders works well most of the time or changes in the conceptual framework would have been made long ago. It is obvious, however, that a Western medical perspective can greatly enhance a Chinese medical understanding of liver/gallbladder function and imbalance in both theory and practice. It may not be enough to diagnose some disorders solely in terms of a Chinese medical perspective. For instance, there are a variety of common diseases which, from a Western medical perspective, must be differentiated from gallbladder disease and which may present very similar Chinese medical signs and symptoms, such as biliary or hepatic types of ulcer distress.[18] The respective Chinese medical diagnosis in this case might conceivably be identical. However, in the case of cholecystitis/cholelithiasis, an additional treatment principle of dissolving stones (if they are present) should be added. While most individuals seeking Chinese medical advice will likely have previously consulted an allopathic physician and will thus present themselves with Western diagnosis in hand, we cannot always count on this to be the case. If one suspects gallbladder disease, it is wise to refer the patient to an allopathic physician for confirmatory diagnosis.

---

18 Ibid., p. 853

While the fundamental diagnosis in the following cases was made according to Chinese medical principles, it is evident that a Western medical understanding has been incorporated into the approach. While concepts of depression, dampness, heat, and stasis-ecchymosis are still primary, and the liver is the primary organ involved, principles such as that of dissolving stones constitute a refinement of therapeutic approach which Chinese medical methodology alone does not provide since there is no way of which I am aware to diagnose gallstones in the Chinese medical framework. Although not all the treatment principles elucidated in the above prescriptions include a specific principle for transforming stones, examination of the prescriptions themselves reveals that they most often include stone-dissolving ingredients. The practitioners were clearly aware of the calculi, and that awareness was facilitated by Western diagnostic methods. For example, in case #7 where there are no calculi shown to be present, this finding is instrumental in shifting the emphasis from that of dissolving calculi to that of dispelling stasis, since this case was of longstanding nature.

Fully one-third of the individuals shown to have gallstones by Western medical tests are totally asymptomatic and, as such, they are often left untreated by Western practitioners.[19] Nonetheless, gallstones are the most frequent cause of gallbladder disease in the long run, particularly among the most common sufferers, characterized by those who are "female, fat, and forty." Certainly it is only logical to address biliary calculi and treat them within the context of a preventative treatment regime. Thus we see the importance of treating the gallbladder as an entity unto itself within the context of a comprehensive Chinese herbal treatment plan.

---

[19] Ibid., p. 853

Arriving at a pattern discrimination [*bian zheng*] for any illness actually represents only a partial diagnosis. A determination of the specific illness involved [*bian bing*] is essential for clarity in an overall treatment plan. *Bian zheng* is the warp and *bian bing* is the woof in the fabric of the diagnostic process. Pattern discrimination is a forte of the TCM paradigm; while *bian bing*, the definition of the specific illness or pathogen, is what modern Western medicine is really all about. Within the context of lung disorders for instance, traditional disease categories such as cough and expectoration, wheezing and dyspnea, pulmonary abscess, pulmonary distension, and pulmonary taxation may all have similar pattern discriminations. Yet, because they are recognized as discrete disease entities, the prescriptions used and the treatment plans employed vary widely from disease to disease. While some *bian bing* are more symptomatic, such as palpitations or chest pain, it is here that refinements based on a modern Western differential diagnosis can augment the clarity of the clinical picture. As can be seen from the previous discussions and the following cases, a wide range of gallbladder disease falls within the traditional categories of costal pain and liver and stomach qi pain. Nonetheless, a significant amount of therapeutic fine tuning can be achieved if a precise Western *bian bing* is ascertained and appended to the overall TCM diagnosis. It is also clear from the previous discussions that, to a greater or lesser extent, the modern Western disease category of cholecystitis is treated as a distinct Chinese medical *bian bing*.

Theoretical Discussions

1. Li Ming-zhen

Cholecyctitis and cholelithiasis in their acute expressions will always be accompanied by costal-abdominal pain and soreness (twisting pain in the gallbladder) [in keeping with the axiom] "where there is pain there is an absence of free flow" [*tong ze bu tong*]. The guiding principle of treatment revolves around the word [*tong*], which can be elaborated to mean "where there is free flow there is no pain" [*tong ze bu tong*]. This is a major principle and cannot be underplayed in draining and purgation to promote free flow of the bowels. Patients will commonly report that their pain diminishes with an episode of diarrhea. If [the condition] can be soothed and drained, then the pain will be greatly diminished, and if it cannot be drained downward, then it is difficult to relieve the pain and soreness. A modification of ***Da Chai Hu Tang*** is most often employed, based upon a combined *shao yang, yang ming* pattern identification, and heavy use of Radix Et Rhizoma Rhei (*Da Huang*) to promote free flow downward yields good results. However, Radix Et Rhizoma Rhei compounds are bitter and difficult to swallow in patients suffering from nausea and vomiting which makes it difficult to give full reign to its medicinal potential. In these instances combined administration of 100 milligrams of powdered raw Semen Crotonis (*Ba Dou*) (approximately one half of one seed) with the decoction will avoid or control any nausea and vomiting. Semen Crotonis also guides and drains and is typically quite effective. If, after 4 hours of administration of the medicinals, no discharge of stool is observed, then another dose may be administered as 4-5 daily watery bowel movements are indicated. Once there is free flow within the bowels and the nausea has been arrested, modifications to ***Da Chai Hu Tang*** can easily be made which will make it easier for the patient to take. The pathomechanism of repletion heat in the liver/gallbladder can also be synthesized [into the prescription]. Some might say, if Semen Crotonis is pungent and warm and then is used to treat patterns of repletion heat in the interior, isn't this like adding fuel to the fire? The error here is in a failure to understand that the nature of Semen Crotonis leans toward harsh and vigorous descension. It functions to completely chop down the gate to the mountain pass and strongly drains repletion. Used in repletion cold its effect is like beating a drum, *i.e.*, it has no purpose in and of itself. Although [Crotonis] treats repletion heat, it specifically pertains to a binding repletion which then generates heat. The implication in promoting free flow is that once the repletion pathogen has been purged, the heat has no place to reside and may then be easily cleared and resolved. This instance of removing the firewood from beneath the cauldron is nothing new. Clinically it is important to make sure that daily dosages not exceed 400 milligrams per day and that ample fluids are provided as well. On the contrary, if one is overcautious and indecisive and hesitates to move forward, one will bungle the case and it will be difficult to achieve a rapid effect. Animal experiments make it clear that Radix Et Rhizoma Rhei and Semen Crotonis both function to disinhibit the gallbladder and are beneficial in removing obstructions from the biliary tract.

2. Hu Jian-hua

It is my feeling that "promoting free flow" [*tong*] is the most common measure employed in the treatment of this illness. It is not, however, the only base therapy. It is sometimes essential go the other way around and, thus, prescription measures for supplementation are employed in the course of therapy. As this illness [cholecystitis] will linger if not cured, it may ultimately recur many times. Clinically, ***Da Chai Hu Tang, [Da] Cheng Qi Tang***, and ***Yin Chen Hao Tang*** are commonly used to clear heat, disinhibit the gallbladder, promote free flow of the bowels, and repeatedly attack [the pathogenic influence]. These prescriptions may, however, ultimately injure the correct qi. If the capacity for the body to heal is weakened, then illnesses will be more frequent, and, if illnesses are more frequent, then this will weaken the capacity of the body to heal. This, then, engenders a vicious cycle, whereby the patient becomes stuck in their suffering. As a result of this, when a condition is resolving slowly, the key to treatment is the emphasis on the word supplementation.

For example, a relatively obese 45 year old female patient had suffered from chronic cholecystitis for ten years, experiencing 5-6 acute episodes a year. Doctors had often used raw Radix Et Rhizoma Rhei in treatment in order to promote free flow and disinhibition. In addition to the above, the patient ordinarily observed a strict diet and had essentially been a vegetarian throughout the year. Therefore, she had a somber, white facial complexion and her essence spirit was faded. She had little appetite, and her dreams were tumultuous and confused. These primary symptoms were those of a vacuity of heart and spleen. She typically tended to urgent right costal distension and pain, radiating up the right side to the shoulder and spine which caused profound suffering. The pulse was fine and weak, lacking strength, while examination of the tongue showed it to be pale and fat. Radix Codonopsis Pilosulae (*Dang Shen*), Radix Astragali Seu Hedysari (*Huang Qi*), Sclerotium Poriae Cocoris (*Fu Ling*), Radix Praeparatus Glycyrrhizae (*Zhi Gan Cao*), were used to supplement the qi and strengthen the spleen. Radix Angelicae Sinensis (*Dang Gui*), Radix Salvia Miltorrhizae (*Dan Shen*), Radix Albus Paeoniae Lactiflorae (*Bai Shao*), Fructus Lycii Chinensis (*Gou Qi Zi*), and Semen Zizyphi Spinosae (*Zao Ren*) were used to nourish the blood, soften the liver, and calm the spirit. These were assisted by Radix Bupleuri (*Chai Hu*), Herba Desmodii Styracofolii (*Jin Qian Cao*), and Radix Et Rhizoma Polygonati Cuspidati (*Hu Chang*) in the class of medicinals which course the liver and disinhibit the gallbladder. Aside from counselling her to adopt a low fat diet, stringent dietary restrictions were not terribly important. With therapy, her facial complexion gradually moistened, her spirits rose, and the costal pain disappeared. She was then given *Gui Pi Tang* as the foundational prescription with the deletions of Arillus Euphoriae Longanae (*Long Yan Rou*), Rhizoma Recens Zingeberis (*Sheng*

Jiang), and Fructus Zizyphii Jujubae (*Da Zao*), and with the additions of Radix Bupleuri (*Chai Hu*), Fructus Citri Seu Ponciri (*Zhi Ke*), Tuber Curcumae (*Yu Jin*), and Fructus Meliae Toosendanis (*Chuan Lian Zi*). This was combined with Colla Cornu Cervi (*Lu Jiao Jiao*) and Saccharum Crystallinum [rock candy] which had been cooked into a paste during the winter to promote supplementation. With continued recuperation over a period of a year, not only was there no recurrence of the frequent costal pain but there were no acute episodes [of cholecystitis] either. Her strength improved daily and she was like a different person at the end [of therapy]. As a result of this, it is my feeling that in the treatment of chronic cholecystitis one cannot obstinately embrace [the axiom] "The six bowels fulfil their purposes when there is free flow [*liu fu yi tong wei yong*]". When integrated with appropriate pattern identification, supplementation may replace purgation. At the same time, if longstanding illness is not cured, the liver channel will become depleted. The softening of the liver should be emphasized as the liver/gallbladderhave a mutual interior/exterior relationship. When the liver is softened and harmonized, the gallbladder qi flows freely and descends, thus the illness is cured of it's own accord.

3. Lin Zong-guang

The following points should be understood in the treatment of cholecystitis:

1. During the acute phase, [measures for] coursing the liver and disinhibiting the gallbladder, clearing, transforming, and promoting free flow downward are indicated for treatment. The joint use of ***Da Chai Hu Tang*** and modified ***Da Xian Xiong Tang*** will resolve it. Radix Bupleuri (*Chai Hu*) 10 grams, prepared Rhizoma Pinelliae Ternatae (*Ban Xia*) 10 gr., Radix Scutellariae Baicalensis (*Huang Qin*) 10 gr., Rhizoma Coptidis Chinensis

(*Huang Lian*) 56 gr., Radix Saussureae Seu Vladimiriae (*Mu Xiang*) 10 gr., Fructus Citri Seu Ponciri (*Zhi Ke*) 10 gr., powdered Rhizoma Corydalis Yanhusuo (*Yan Hu Suo*) 10-15 gr., raw Radix Et Rhizoma Rhei (*Da Huang*) 10-12 gr., and Herba Artemesiae Capillaris (*Yin Chen*) 10 gr. are most commonly used, modified according to the symptoms. Following administration of the medicinals, [the patient] should have 2-4 bowel movements a day, which should rapidly reduce the heat/fever and cause the abdominal pain to gradually disappear. A small number of patients will have some residual right subcostal distension, poor appetite, or a mild degree of right subcostal pressure pain. In this case the prescription is shifted to the use of ***Xiao Yao San*** and/or modified ***Da Xian Xiong Tang***. Medicinals such as Radix Bupleuri, Radix Albus Paeoniae Lactiflorae, Radix Saussureae Seu Vladimiriae, Fructus Citri Seu Ponciri, Tuber Curcumae, and powdered Rhizoma Corydalis Yanhusuo are then added.

2. During the inactive phase, the clinical manifestations are most often atypical, and [the patient] may even be asymptomatic. The following types, however, are seen relatively often:

A. There may be non-specific manifestations in the gastro-intestinal tract such as diminished appetite, post-prandial gastric distension, lack of strength, dull facial complexion, and a thin, wiry pulse. In this case [measures for] coursing the liver and disinhibiting the gallbladder, purging the interior and promoting free flow downward are indicated. 10 grams each of Radix Bupleuri, Radix Saussureae Seu Vladimiriae, Fructus Citri Seu Ponciri, Tuber Curcumae, and powdered Rhizoma Corydalis Yanhusuo with modifications are typically used. If the tongue moss is slimy and yellow, there is a bitter taste in the mouth, and there is dark urine, then add Herba Artemesiae Capillaris, Herba Desmodii Styracifolii (*Jin Qian Cao*), and Rhizoma Coptidis Chinensis. If the tongue moss is slimy and white, then add prepared Rhizoma Pinelliae Ternatae and Cortex Magnoliae

Officinalis (*Hou Po*). If there is spleen vacuity, add Radix Codonopsis Pilosulae (*Dang Shen*) and Rhizoma Atractylodis Macrocephalae (*Bai Zhu*). Administration of these medicinals will maintain smooth bowel movements 1-2 times a day with daily improvement.

B. If the patient presents as asymptomatic with "symptoms of a normal person" or in conjunction with a gall stone pattern, then the prescription should be composed of Radix Bupleuri 10 gr., Radix Saussureae Seu Vladimiriae 10 gr., Fructus Citri Seu Ponciri 10 gr., Tuber Curcumae 10 gr., and 10 grams each powdered Rhizoma Corydalis Yanhusuo, and Herbae Artemesiae Capillaris , 5 doses administered as a course. Persevering in therapy will then guard against recurrences. In addition, since Chinese medical theory suggests that chronic stasis of the liver and gallbladder qi may take the form of blood stasis, two or three medicinals such as Semen Pruni Persicae (*Tao Ren*), Radix Salviae Miltorrhizae (*Dan Shen*), and Radix Albus Paeoniae Lactiflorae may be added to the prescriptions mentioned above.

4. Li Xue-zheng

Based on clinically seen patterns, chronic cholecystitis falls within the scope of costal pain, liver and stomach qi pain, and liver/gallbaldder disease in Chinese medicine. The *Zhang Lun Pian* in the *Nei Jing* states: "Liver distension is subcostal fullness and pain radiating to the lateral umbilical area", and, "Gallbladder distension is subcostal distension and pain". Clinically, the pattern discrimination falls largely into patterns of depressive binding of liver qi and dampness and heat in liver and gallbladder with disharmony between liver and stomach. The treatment measures for this illness are to purge the interior and promote free flow downward, clear heat and resolve poisons, rectify the qi, open depression, and disinhibit the gallbladder. For qi stasis and depressive heat in the liver and gallbladder, ***Si Ni Tang*** and ***Da***

Chai Hu Tang are indicated. Medicinal substances such as Radix Bupleuri, Radix Albus Paeoniae Lactiflorae, Radix Scutellariae Baicalensis, Cortex Radicis Moutan (*Dan Pi*), Fructus Gardeniae Jasminoidis (*Zhi Zi*), Radix Et Rhizoma Rhei, and Radix Glycyrrhizae (*Gan Cao*) are commonly used. For obstructive dampness and heat in the liver and gallbladder, ***Yin Chen Hao Tang*** and ***Long Dan Xie Gan Tang*** are indicated. Medicinals such as Herba Artemesiae Capillaris, Fructus Gardeniae Jasminoidis, Radix Scutellariae Baicalensis, Radix Bupleuri, Radix Gentiana Scabrae (*Long Dan Cao*), Caulis Akebiae Mutong (*Mu Tong*), Semen Plantaginis (*Che Qian Zi*), Rhizoma Alismatis (*Ze Xie*), Radix Et Rhizoma Rhei, and Radix Glycyrrhizae are used [in this case]. If [the cholecystitis] is due to an acute parasite, use ***Wu Mei An Hui Tang***, the components of which include Fructus Pruni Mume (*Wu Mei*), Rhizoma Coptidis Chinensis, Cortex Phellodendri (*Huang Bai*), Fructus Zanthoxyli Bungeanae (*Chuan Jiao*), Herba Cum Radice Asari Sieboldi (*Xi Xin*), Fructus Meliae Toosendanis, Radix Angelicae Sinensis, Radix Albus Paeoniae Lactiflorae, Tuber Curcumae, and Radix Glycyrrhizae.

Radix Bupleuri is not the least of the medicinals in prescriptions for coursing the liver and resolving depression mentioned above. In addition, the promotion of free flow is primary in the treatment of chronic cholecystitis, and Radix Et Rhizoma Rhei does not fall short as a useful medicinal for this purpose. It is capable of draining heat and transforming stasis, and achieves quite a rapid effect when used for patterns of depressive heat.

Case histories

Case 1: Cholecystitis

Zhao Di-hua

Chinese medical pattern discrimination: Stasis of liver/gallbladder qi, internal depression of dampness and heat

Treatment measures: Course the liver and disinhibit the gallbladder, rectify the qi and relieve depression, clear and transform dampness and heat

Prescription: *Xin Qing Dan Tang*

Ingredients:

raw Radix Astragali Seu Hedysari (*Huang Qi*) 31g
Herba Desmodii Styrachifolii (*Jin Qian Cao*) 62g
Radix Bupleuri (*Chai Hu*) 12-24g
Radix Albus Paeoniae Lactiflorae (*Bai Shao*) 12-15g
Tuber Curcumae (*Yu Jin*) 12g
Herba Cum Radice Taraxaci Mongolici (*Pu Gong Ying*) 24-31g
Rhizoma Corydalis Yanhusuo (*Yan Hu Suo*) 9-12g
Herba Oldenlandiae Diffusae (*Bai Hua She She Cao*) 31g
Radix Dioscoreae Oppositae (*Shan Yao*) 24g
Endothelium Corneum Gigeraiae Galli (*Ji Nei Jin*) 9-12g

This is [for] one day; a course of therapy is 20 doses.

If the patient is weak with qi vacuity, increase the Radix Astragali Seu Hedysari to 64 gr. If the patient suffers from diaphoresis add Fructus Levis Tritici (*Fu Xiao Mai*) 31-62g and Radix Ephedrae (*Ma Huang Gen*) 12g. If the patient suffers from blood vacuity, add Caulis Milletiae Seu Spatholobi (*Ji Xue Teng*) 24g. In the event that there is no qi depression with abdominal pain, delete Rhizoma Corydalis Yanhusuo. If there is nausea and vomiting, add Rhizoma Pinelliae Ternatae, and Caulis Bambusae

In Taeniis (*Zhu Ru*). With constipation, add wine-treated Radix Et Rhizoma Rhei and, with abdominal distension and pain, add Miribilitum (*Mang Xiao*).

Case: A 36 year old female medical technician had one year previously experienced an episode of acute cholecystitis accompanied by a low-grade fever. There were many symptoms which were yang in nature. The pulse was wiry and slippery and her tongue moss was thin and yellow. She was given ***Xing Qing Dan Tang*** and all her symptoms disappeared. She finished the course of medication one month later and, when contacted 11 years later, she reported that she had experienced no recurrence.

Case 2: Cholecystitis (During Pregnancy)

Wu Cheng-zhong

Chinese medical pattern discrimination: Pain in the branch connecting vessel of the heart during pregnancy.

Treatment principle: Transform dampness and heat in order to clear it internally, warm the qi of the channels and disperse it externally, rectify the qi and blood, and rid soreness and pain

Prescription: ***Huo Long San*** with additions.

Ingredients:

stir-fried Fructus Meliae Toosendanis (*Chuan Lian Zi*) 9g
stir-fried Fructus Foeniculi Vulgaris (*Xiao Hui Xiang*) 9g
Folium Artemisiae Argyii (*Ai Ye*) stir-fried in salt water, 4.5g
Radix Bupleuri (*Chai Hu*) 3g
Radix Scutellariae Baicalensis (*Huang Qin*) 4.5g

Decocted in water, this is one *ji.*[20]

Case: A 36 year old housewife was admitted to the hospital for treatment complaining of pain and fullness in the chest and gastric cavity. She was diagnosed as suffering from cholecystitis. The medical treatment she received yielded no outstanding results, and on May 8, 1950, she returned for further diagnosis. The patient presented with intermittent chest and gastric pain and her body was alternately chilled and feverish. Her tongue moss was thick, charred black, and slightly yellow. When her pain stopped, the moss would gradually recede and the chills and fever would abate. Conversely, when the pain intensified, the signs and symptoms would return. She was five months pregnant and presented a wiry, somewhat rapid pulse. It is recognized in Chinese medicine that the heart is the sovereign and, as such, cannot be attacked by external pathogens. This role of receiving attack falls to the heart connecting vessel, causing a disruption in equanimity and heart pain, thus the diagnosis of pain in the branch *luo* of the heart during pregnancy. Because of the fever and chills accompanying the pain, ***Xin Qing Dan Tang*** with additions was employed. Two doses were administered and the pain promptly ceased, as did the chills and fever. The charred, yellow moss also retreated. Radix Bupleuri and Radix Scutellariae Baicalensis were deleted from the prescription and two more doses were administered to consolidate the treatment effect. With no more pain, she recovered fully and was discharged. In the spring of 1951, the patient reported that she had experienced no recurrence of the illness. She gave birth to a plump and healthy child.

---

20 The word *ji* literally means formula. It cannot be translated accurately as either dose, packet, day's supply, or any other term. Since translating it literally as formula seems confusing in English, we have chosen to leave it in Chinese pinyin.

Case 3: Chronic Cholecystitis and Acute Cholelithiasis

Su Li

Chinese medical pattern discrimination: Stasis and depression of liver and gallbladder

Treatment measures: Course the liver, disinhibit the gallbladder, transform stasis and stop pain (in the acute manifestation); regulate the qi, harmonize the blood, benefit the stomach, and disperse stagnation (in the chronic manifestation)

Prescriptions: *Qing Dan Tang* (for the acute manifestation); *Chuan Lian Zi San* (for the chronic manifestation).

***Qing Dan Tang* ingredients:**

Radix Bupleuri (*Chai Hu*) 12g
Radix Scutellariae Baicalensis (*Huang Qin*) 10g
Rhizoma Pinelliae Ternatae (*Ban Xia*) 10g
Radix Albus Paeoniae Lactiflorae (*Bai Shao*) 12g
Radix Et Rhizoma Rhei (*Da Huang*) added afterward, 12g
Fructus Citri Seu Ponciri (*Zhi Ke*) 12g
Rhizoma Corydalis Yanhusuo (*Yuan Hu*) 10g
Radix Saussureae Seu Vladimiriae (*Mu Xiang*) 10g
Herba Lycopi Lucidi (*Ze Lan*) 12g
Rhizoma Recens Zingiberis (*Sheng Jiang*) 6g
Fructus Zizyphi Jujubae (*Da Zao*) 3 pieces
Radix Pseudoginseng (*San Qi*) crushed, 5g

Decocted in water, one dose is administered daily. (If necessary one may take two doses four times a day.)

***Chuan Lian Zi San* ingredients:**

fried Fructus Meliae Toosendanis (*Chuan Lian Zi*) 30g
Rhizoma Corydalis Yanhusuo (*Yan Hu Suo*) cooked in vinegar, 30 g.
Tuber Curcumae (*Yu Jin*) 60g
Herba Cyn Radice Taraxici Mongolici (*Pu Gong Ying*) 60g
Endothelium Corneum Gigierae Galli (*Ji Nei Jin*) 30g

Finely grind up the constituents, take six grams 3-4 times a day; a course of therapy is three months.

Comment: Satisfactory results were obtained in clinical use of the above two prescriptions in over 100 cases. In general, approximately three doses of ***Qing Dan Tang*** will control the symptoms, while afterward the use of ***Chuan Lian Zi San*** through 1-3 courses of therapy will gradually reduce the patient's symptoms, resulting in a complete cure.

Case: A 50 year old woman habitually suffered from "heartburn" which had been occurring 2-3 times a month for the past ten years. With each episode she would experience violent soreness and pain causing her to double up and hold her abdomen as she tossed and turned, with pain radiating into the shoulder and spine, nausea and vomiting, and a drenching cold sweat. At a hospital, she was diagnosed as suffering from chronic cholecystitis and acute cholelithiasis. She had frequently used antibiotics and atropine preparations but with poor results.

When the patient was diagnosed, the acute symptomology was prevalent. The major symptoms were the same as above but also included dry stools, yellow-red urine, a red tongue with thick, yellow moss, a tense, wiry pulse and relatively yellow sclera. The diagnosis was depression and stagnancy of the liver/gallbladder.

Qing Dan Tang was prescribed. After one dose the pain diminished, and following three doses all symptoms disappeared. Following this, ***Chuan Lian Zi San*** was administered. During the course of treatment, she only suffered two attacks and the intensity of the episodes was greatly decreased. During the first course, she felt no more gastric and abdominal upset, the dispersing function increased her appetite, and she felt no trace of the illness. In the three years since she finished the medication, she has had no recurrence of the problem.

Case 4: Cholelithiasis

Weng Nan-gong

Chinese medical pattern discrimination: Depressive binding of liver qi, depression of wood transforming to fire

Treatment measures: Course the liver and regulate the qi, clear heat and transform stasis, disinhibit the gallbladder and expel stones

Prescription: ***Qing Dan Hua Shi Tang***

Ingredients:

Radix Bupleuri (*Chai Hu*) 6g
Herba Hydrocotylis (*Man Tian Xing*) 15g
Rhizoma Corydalis Yanhusuo (*Yan Hu Suo*) 6g
Herba Desmodii Styrachifolii (*Jin Qian Cao*) 15g
Fructus Meliae Toosendanis (*Chuan Lian Zi*) 9g
Radix Scutellariae Baicalensis (*Huang Qin*) 9g
Tuber Curcumae (*Yu Jin*) 6g

Medulla Tetrapanacis Papyriferi (*Tong Cao*) 3g
Herba Cum Radice Taraxaci Mongolici (*Pu Gong Ying*) 12g
northern Herba Artemesiae Capillaris (*Yin Chen Hao*) 15g

Decocted in water, one dose is taken daily.

Case: A 54 year old male worker was first examined on October 8, 1974. He had suffered from an oppressive pain in his upper abdominal region, which at times was acute, for many years. It was most often sore and painful after the midday meal but had recently become a continual dull pain and had gradually begun to radiate acutely into the shoulder area, with intolerably profuse perspiration. One month previously, he had been admitted to a hospital and was diagnosed as having gallstones. After receiving therapy, he was discharged but the problem returned with frequent bitter taste in the mouth, nausea, vomiting and lack of appetite, abdominal distention, and urination which was short and dark. The abdomen was painful to palpation. There was no jaundice, the tip of the tongue was red, and there was a thick yellow moss on it. The pulse in the left *guan* position was wiry and urgent; while the right *guan* position was wiry and rapid. The Chinese medical diagnosis was depression of liver qi, depression of wood transforming into fire. Treatment measures were to course the liver, regulate the qi, clear heat, transform stasis, disinhibit the gallbladder, and discharge stones. The patient took six doses of ***Qing Dan Hua Shi Tan*** and the rib pain was greatly reduced, as was the severity of his pain in general. The left pulse was wiry and rapid, while the right became wiry and thin. The tongue was red with thin, yellow moss and the urination became somewhat long. All [these] indicated that the liver qi had been coursed and the fire quelled. He continued the above prescription for four more doses, after which the pain completely disappeared. There remained some epigastric oppression and soreness and lack of appetite. He had a wiry left pulse and a thin right pulse, while the tongue was red with a white moss. This indicated that the spleen was being injured by wood. Thus the prescription for rectifying the liver qi was modified to strengthen the spleen and transform dampness.

Cortex Magnoliae Officinalis (*Hou Po*) 9g
Sclerotium Poriae Cocoris (*Fu Ling*) 9g
Fructus Meliae Toosendanis (*Chuan Lian Zi*) was reduced to 9g;
Radix Albus Peoniae Lactiflorae (*Bai Shao*) 9g
Fructus Germinatus Hordei Vulgaris (*Mai Ya*) 9g
Radix Saussureae Seu Vladimiriae (*Mu Xiang*) 6g
Radix Gentianae Scabrae (*Long Dan Cao*) 6g
Radix Codonopsis Pilosulae (*Dang Shen*) 12g

One month later the patient was x-rayed again and the stones in the biliary tract were no longer present. Following five more doses, the appetite returned and the epigastric distention also diminished.

Comment: ***Qing Dan Hua Shi Tang*** has been employed time and again in cases of acute cholelithiasis. Herba Hydrocotylis as used in the prescription has a strong effect in disinhibiting the gallbladder and expelling stones.

Cases 5 & 6: Cholecystitis and Cholelithiasis

Xie Xin-jian

Chinese medical discrimination of patterns: Liver depression and qi stasis

Treatment measures: Course the liver and relieve depression, rectify the qi and arrest pain

Prescription: ***Shu Gan Li Dan Tang (Wan)***

Ingredients:

Radix Bupleuri (*Chai Hu*) 10g
Fructus Citri Seu Ponciri (*Zhi Ke*) 10g
Pericarpium Viridis Citri Reticulatae (*Qing Pi*) 10g
Pericarpium Citri Reticulatae (*Chen Pi*) 10g
Rhizoma Et Radix Polygonati Cuspidati (*Hu Chang*) 30g
Flos Lonicerae Japonicae (*Jin Ying Hua*) 30g
Radix Et Rhizoma Rhei (*Da Huang*) 12g
Mirabilitum (*Mang Xiao*) 10g
Herba Desmodii Styrachifolii (*Jin Qian Cao*) 30g
Herba Artemesiae Capillaris (*Yin Chen Hao*) 30g
Tuber Curcumae (*Yu Jin*) 12g
Fructus Meliae Toosendanis (*Chuan Lian Zi*) 12g
Rhizoma Corydalis Yanhusuo (*Yan Hu Suo*) 10g
Radix Albus Paeoniae Lactiflorae (*Bai Shao*) 12g

Decocted in water, one *ji* is taken daily.

Dosage for pills: Finely grind all the ingredients and mix with water into pills more or less the size of *Wu Tong* seeds (Chinese parasol fruits) taking 50-60 each time with warm boiled water 2-3 times a day.

Comment: Clinical practice demonstrates that ***Shu Gan Li Dan Tang (Wan)*** is clinically superior in definitively disinhibiting the gallbladder and clearing inflammation. In ten cases, it has been successful in avoiding surgical intervention when the prescription was used daily and with perseverance. In acute episodes it is appropriate to use the prescription in decoction; while in cases of chronic illness or in patients with both acute and chronic expression of the illness the use of pill form is indicated.

Case 5: A 50 year old woman was first seen on June 26, 1977. She was experiencing acute right upper abdominal pain, nausea, vomiting, fear of chill, and a fever. She was diagnosed as having an acute attack of chronic cholecystitis compounded with both an obstruction and inflammation of the bile duct. Several years prior during an attack, her liver/gallbladdercondition had been reliably diagnosed as cholecystitis and cholelithiasis. In the previous two years, she had suffered frequent episodes where she was unable to work, and in the last year she had entirely stopped doing any housework. This time when she was admitted to the hospital, surgery was recommended. However, the patient refused this option and the situation was managed using a conservative Western pharmacological therapy. This combatted the inflammation and disinhibited the gallbladder following an entire course of therapy with a number of drugs. Although the disease process abated taking a positive turn, the acute right upper abdominal pain persisted as did her lack of appetite. She continued to have a bitter taste in her mouth and a dry throat. Though thirsty, she lacked a desire to drink. She was cold with chilled extremities, was constipated, and her urine was yellow. Her body temperature was 38.2° Celsius and she presented with a wiry pulse, a slimy, yellow tongue moss with a red tip, and her sclera and skin were slightly yellow. The diagnosis was liver depression and qi stagnation with dampness and heat accumulating on the interior. Therefore, ***Shu Gan Li Dan Tang*** was prescribed. Following the administration of three doses all the symptoms were distinctly diminished. The patient was instructed to take another four doses and following this all her symptoms disappeared. She related that her bowel movements were slightly watery and somewhat more frequent. Her prescription was changed to pill form which she continued to take for two more years. She returned to work and continued working full time for a year and eleven months and at that time had no recurrence of her illness.

Case 6: A 52 year old male was first examined on July 16, 1977. The patient had undergone surgery for gallstones the year before and had currently been admitted to the hospital for residual stones in the biliary tract. He had been recommended for surgery twice to eliminate the stones, though he had refused and elected to try an herbal therapy. The patient presented with acute and severe upper right quadrant abdominal pain accompanied by a dry, bitter taste in his mouth, lack of appetite, yellow urine, and a yellow tongue moss. His diagnosis was liver depression and qi stasis and ***Shu Gan Li Dan Wan*** was administered.

On May 10, 1980, the patient reported that after taking the above prescription there had been no recurrence of liver and gallbladder problems and that it was only when he was very busy working and forgot to take his medicine for several days that he would feel somewhat out of sorts. However, within a half hour of resuming his medication all the symptoms would vanish.

Case 7: Chronic biliary infection cholangitis.

Mai Guan-min

Chinese medical pattern discrimination: Stasis of qi and blood

Treatment measures: Course the liver, rectify the qi, circulate blood stasis, and disperse jaundice.

Prescription: ***Chai Hu Wu Chu Tang***

Ingredients:

Radix Bupleuri (*Chai Hu*) 12g

Radix Albus Paeoniae Lactiflorae (*Bai Shao*) 12g
Pericarpium Citri Reticulatae (*Chen Pi*) 10g
Radix Pseudostellariae Heterophyllae (*Tai Zi Shen*) 30g
Rhizoma Curcumae Zedoariae (*E Zhu*) 12g

Decocted in water, one dose is taken daily

With a red tongue and a yellow cast [to the complexion] one may add Herba Desmodii Styrachifolii, Herba Artemesia Capillaris, and Radix Et Rhizoma Rhei.

Case: A 34 year old female worker was first examined on January 10, 1976. Ten years previously the patient had undergone a cholecystectomy due to the presence of biliary calculi, after which she frequently experienced a fear of cold and a fever accompanied by right upper abdominal discomfort, yellow eyes, and yellow skin. However, each time she underwent treatment to clear the heat and disinhibit the gallbladder, the therapy was of no lasting benefit and the problem would inevitably return. Her tongue was pale with white moss and she presented with a wiry pulse. Her upper abdominal areas were not particularly painful to palpation. A contrast medium of the bile duct showed no stones; thus, the diagnosis was stasis-ecchymosis of the gallbladder collaterals which were not being cleaned. ***Chai Hu Wu Chu Tang*** was administered and she took seven doses, after which her pain completely disappeared while her other symptoms were greatly diminished. The patient was discharged from the hospital, and, after taking many more doses of the medication, was completely cured. In a follow-up call a number of years later she reported no recurrence of the symptoms.

Comment: There are categories of yin jaundice which are divided between the *zang* and the *fu*. It has been said that, "Jaundice generally comes under the category of dampness and heat." One should know that, "In the illnesses of the 100 vessels, obstructed heat exists internally." One's color thus will be seen to be yellow. Dampness and heat accumulate in the blood, but treating the problem with substances of a bitter and cold nature is inappropriate for relieving the obstruction. It is an unspoken principle that, in order to treat jaundice, one must first treat the blood; when the blood moves, the jaundice is vanquished of its own accord.

The methodology for moving stasis and ridding jaundice is well documented. To rectify the qi and move the blood, a combination of salty, descending, and warm and penetrating ingredients should be used to treat gallstones, as this has been tested and proven time and again. Our ancestors have sated that "The more chronic the disease, the greater the stasis-ecchymosis". With respect to cases of intractable illness, this concept of stasis-ecchymosis is of great relevance. Therefore, many *bian zheng* employ the above principle as a foundation, giving emphasis to moving the blood and transforming stasis-ecchymosis by using substances which regulate the blood and thus they achieve good results.

HOT UNDER THE COLLAR

Distinguished Physicians Discuss the Treatment of Hypertension

Introduction

This chapter contains the essays of six eminent practitioners of Chinese herbal medicine on the treatment of hypertension followed by three case histories. Virtually all of these physicians describe hyperactivity of liver fire, often with attendant vacuity of kidney yin, as the most common pattern of this illness. Nonetheless, the particulars of diagnosis and treatment are idiosyncratic to each individual practitioner. Tan Ri-xiang divides hypertension into three patterns of hyperactive ascension of liver yang, internal accumulation of phlegm heat, and vacuity of liver and kidney yin. Chen Shu-sen advocates lifestyle modifications in 70% of his hypertension patients as a means of treating the disease and prescribes medication in only 30% of his patients. Wu Gong-song prefers to employ modifications of *Xi Feng Tang* in his therapy. While Zhu Gu-ting treats hypertension based on tongue differentiations. Wei Zhang-chun prefers prescriptions of his own formulation in the treatment of hypertension and, finally, Chen Ze-lin discusses the importance of combining *bian zheng* and *bian bing* to achieve successful results in the treatment of hypertension. The essays of Tan Ri-xiang, Chen Shu-sheng, Wu Song-kang, and Zhu Gu-ting are translated in full. Those of Wei Zhang-chun and Chen Ze-lin contain much of the same material as the above four and so only material unique to their respective approaches has been included.

Tan Ri-xiang [I]

The clinical manifestations of hypertension can be divided into three syndromes for treatment.

1. Ascending hyperactivity of liver yang: This is characterized by symptoms of cerebral dizziness, headache, sudden irritability, vexation, and tendency to become easily angered, a bitter taste in the mouth, and facial redness accompanied by a red tongue with yellow fur and a wiry, forceful pulse. It is, therefore, appropriate to clear the liver and restrain the yang. If there is a tendency towards effulgence of liver fire, then use ***Tian Ma Gou Teng Yin***:

Rhizoma Gastrodiae Elatae (*Tian Ma*)
Ramulus Uncariae Cum Uncis (*Gou Teng*)
Fructus Gardeniae Jasminoidis (*Zhi Zi*)
Radix Scutellariae Baicalensis (*Huang Qin*)
Radix Achyranthis Bidentatae (*Niu Xi*)
Caulis Polygoni Multiflori (*Ye Jiao Teng*)
Concha Haliotidis (*Shi Jue Ming*)
Ramus Loranthi Seu Visci (*Sang Ji Sheng*)
Sclerotium Poriae Cocoris (*Fu Ling*)
Cortex Eucommiae Ulmoidis (*Du Zhong*)
Herba Leonuri Heterophylli (*Yi Mu Cao*)

If there is a tendency toward hyperactivity of wind/yang, then use ***Zhen Gan Xi Feng Tang***:

Radix Scrophulariae Ningpoensis (*Yuan Shen*)
Tuber Ophiopogonis Japonicae (*Mai Dong*)
Fructus Meliae Toosendanis (*Chuan Lian Zi*)
Radix Albus Paeoniae Lactiflorae (*Bai Shao*)
Plastrum Testudinis (*Gui Ban*)
Radix Achyranthis Bidentatae (*Niu Xi*)

Hematitum (*Dai Zhe Shi*)
raw Os Draconis (*Sheng Long Gu*)
raw Concha Ostreae (*Sheng Mu Li*)
Herba Artemesiae Capillaris (*Yin Chen*)
Fructus Germinatus Hordei Vulgaris (*Mai Ya*)
Radix Glycyrrhizae (*Gan Cao*)

2. Internal abundance of phlegm fire: This is characterized by symptoms of heavy headedness and vertigo, thoracic oppression, upflow and nausea, vexation and insomnia, a bitter taste in the mouth, and yellow urine accompanied by a yellow, slimy tongue fur and slippery, wiry pulse. It is, therefore, appropriately treated by cleansing phlegm and ridding heat. If the patient is obese, then use ***Gou Teng Wen Dan Tang*** [containing]:

Ramulus Uncariae Cum Uncis (*Gou Teng*)
Flos Chrysanthemi Morifolii (*Ju Hua*)
Fructus Tribuli Terrestris (*Bai Ji Li*)
Rhizoma Pinelliae Ternatae (*Ban Xia*)
Sclerotium Poriae Cocoris (*Fu Ling*)
Pericarpium Citri Reticulatae (*Chen Pi*)
Rhizoma Coptidis Chinensis (*Huang Lian*)
Caulis Bambusae In Taeniis (*Zhu Ru*)
Radix Achyranthis Bidentatae (*Niu Xi*)
Lumbricus (*Di Long*)
Radix Glycyrrhizae (*Gan Cao*)

If the patient has a bony body type, then use ***Ling Jiao Gou Teng Tang***:

Cornu Antelopis (*Ling Yang Jiao*)
Ramulus Uncariae Cum Uncis (*Gou Teng*)
Folium Mori Albi (*Sang Ye*)
Flos Chrysanthemi Morifolii (*Ju Hua*)
Radix Rehmanniae (*Sheng Di*)

Radix Albus Paeoniae Lactiflorae (*Bai Shao*)
Bulbus Fritillariae Thunbergii (*Bei Mu*)
Sclerotium Poriae Cocoris (*Fu Ling*)
Caulis Bambusae In Taeniis (*Zhu Ru*)
Radix Glycyrrhizae (*Gan Cao*)

3. Vacuity of liver and kidney yin: This is characterized by cephalic dizziness, headache, tinnitus and visual dizziness, soreness and feebleness of the lumbus and knees, nocturnal enuresis and seminal emission, all accompanied by a red tongue with little moss and a fine, wiry pulse. It is appropriately treated by enriching the kidneys and softening the liver. If there is a [stronger] tendency toward liver yin vacuity then use ***Shou Wu Yan Shou Dan***:

Radix Polygoni Multiflori (*He Shou Wu*)
Radix Achyranthis Bidentatae (*Niu Xi*)
Semen Cuscutae (*Tu Si Zi*)
Cortex Eucommiae Ulmoidis (*Du Zhong*)
Folium Mori Albi (*Sang Ye*)
Flos Chrysanthemi Morifolii (*Ju Hua*)
Fructus Mori Albi (*Sang Shen*)
Fructus Ligustri Lucidi (*Nu Zhen Zi*)
Herba Ecliptae Prostratae (*Han Lian Cao*)
Semen Sesami (*Hei Zhi Ma*)
Herba Siegesbeckiae (*Xi Jian Cao*)

If there is a [stronger] tendency toward kidney yin vacuity then use ***Qi Ju Di Huang Wan***:

Fructus Lycii Chinensis (*Gou Qi Zi*)
Flos Chrysanthemi Morifolii (*Ju Hua*)
Radix Coquitus Rehmanniae (*Shu Di*)
Rhizoma Curculiginis Orchoidis (*Xian Mao*)
Sclerotium Poriae Cocoris (*Fu Ling*)

Cortex Radicis Moutan (*Dan Pi*)
Rhizoma Alismatis (*Ze Xie*)
Fructus Corni Officinalis (*Shan Zhu Yu*)
Radix Achyranthis Bidentatae (*Niu Xi*)
Plastrum Testudinis (*Gui Ban*)

Using the above three syndromes and six prescriptions in the treatment [of hypertension] a will achieve a positive result.

Chen Shu-sheng [I]

In the clinical treatment of hypertension, I believe that 30% require medication, while 70% require lifestyle modification. The patient should not be nervous or suffer from sudden agitation or anxiety and he should get enough sleep and appropriate amounts of exercise. With respect to diet, fatty, sweet, and salty foods should be avoided in favor of a bland, vegetarian diet. The appetite must be controlled and the patient must gradually lose weight. With respect to herbal therapy, the following should be administered:

In the case of an ascending hyperactivity of liver yang, measures for levelling the liver and restraining the yang should be employed, assisted by measures for nourishing the heart and calming the spirit. I therefore use ***Tian Ma Gou Teng Yin*** with modifications:

Rhizoma Gastrodiae Elatae (*Tian Ma*) 10g
Ramulus Uncariae Cum Uncis (*Gou Teng*) 20g
Flos Chrysanthemi Indici (*Ye Ju Hua*) 15g
Concha Haliotidis (*Shi Jue Ming*) 30g
Radix Scutellariae Baicalensis (*Huang Qin*) 15g
Sclerotium Poriae Cocoris (*Fu Ling*) 15g
Caulis Polygoni Multiflori (*Ye Jiao Teng*) 20g

Spica Prunellae Vulgaris (*Xia Gu Cao*) 15g
Radix Achyranthis Bidentatae (*Niu Xi*) 10g
Rhizoma Anemarrhenae (*Zhi Mu*) 10g
Semen Zizyphi Spinosae (*Zao Ren*) 15g

For ocular redness and yellow urine add:

Radix Gentianae Scabrae (*Long Dan Cao*)
Rhizoma Alismatis (*Ze Xie*)

For constipation and dry stools add:

Semen Cassiae Torae (*Jue Ming Zi*)
Radix Rehmanniae (*Sheng Di*)

In the case of vacuity of yin and hyperactivity of liver yang, measures to enrich the yin and restrain the yang are to be employed, for which I use ***Qi Ju Di Huang Tang*** with modifications:

Fructus Lycii Chinensis (*Gou Qi*) 10g
Flos Chrysanthemi Indici (*Ye Ju Hua*) 15g
Radix Rehmanniae (*Sheng Di*) 15g
Fructus Corni Officinalis (*Shan Zhu Yu*) 9g
Rhizoma Alismatis (*Ze Xie*) 15g
Sclerotium Poriae Cocoris (*Fu Ling*) 15g
Cortex Radicis Moutan (*Dan Pi*) 10g
Radix Achyranthis Bidentatae (*Niu Xi*) 10g
Ramulus Uncariae Cum Uncis (*Gou Teng*) 20g
Ramus Loranthi Seu Visci (*Sang Ji Sheng*) 15g
raw Os Draconis (*Sheng Long Gu*) 15g
raw Concha Ostrea (*Sheng Mu Li*) 15g
Radix Albus Paeoniae Lactiflorae (*Bai Shao*) 15g

If the patient has difficulty falling asleep or is easily awakened, then add:

baked Radix Polygalae Tenufoliae (*Yuan Zhi*)
Semen Zizyphi Spinosae (*Zao Ren*)

and before bed administer *Yuan Ming Fen* 4 g [powder of Radix Glycyrrhizae (*Gan Cao*) treated with sodium sulfate and] artificial Calculus Bovis (*Niu Huang*) 0.5 g

If there is oppressive pain in the precordial area, particularly following exercise, then add:

Radix Salviae Miltiorrhizae (*Dan Shen*)
Rhizoma Ligustici Wallichi (*Chuan Xiong*)
Flos Carthami Tinctorii (*Hong Hua*)

For tension in the suboccipital and cervical region, add:

Radix Puerariae Lobatae (*Ge Gen*)
Rhizoma Ligustici Wallichi (*Chuan Xiong*)

For numbness in the extremities, add:

Herba Siegesbeckiae (*Xi Jian Cao*)
Ramulus Mori Albi (*Sang Zhi*)
Lumbricus (*Di Long*)

For swelling and distension in both lower limbs, add:

Radix Stephaniae Tetandrae (*Han Fang Ji*)
Sclerotium Poriae Cocoris (*Fu Ling*)
Thallus Algae (*Kun Bu*)

In the case of a joint vacuity of yin and yang, then employ measures to enrich the yin and support the yang, level the liver and invigorate the blood, for which ***Jin Gui Shen Qi Wan*** with modification is commonly used:

Radix Coquitus Rehmanniae (*Shu Di*) 15g
Fructus Corni Officinalis (*Shan Zhu Yu*) 10g
Radix Dioscoreae Oppositae (*Shan Yao*) 10g
Sclerotium Poriae Cocoris (*Fu Ling*) 10g
Cortex Radix Moutan (*Dan Pi*) 10g
Rhizoma Alismatis (*Ze Xie*) 10g
Ramulus Uncariae Cum Uncis (*Gou Teng*) 20g
Flos Chrysanthemi Indici (*Ye Ju Hua*) 15g
Herba Epimedii (*Xian Ling Pi*) 15g
Radix Salviae Miltiorrhizae (*Dan Shen*) 15g
Rhizoma Ligustici Wallichii (*Chuan Xiong*) 15g
Herba Sargassi (*Hai Zao*) 15g
Cortex Cinnamomi (*Rou Gui*) 2g

For frequent enuresis, add:

Semen Alpiniae Oxyphyllae (*Yi Zhi Ren*)
Fructus Psoraleae Corylifoliae (*Bu Gu Zhi*)

For spiritual fatigue and lack of strength, add:

Radix Astragali Seu Hedysari (*Huang Qi*)
Radix Codonopsis Pilosulae (*Dang Shen*)

For oppression of the chest, shortness of breath, and palpitations, add:

Tuber Ophiopogonis Japonicae (*Mai Dong*)
Fructus Schizandrae Chinensis (*Wu Wei*)
Radix Panacis Ginseng (*Ren Shen*)

For vexation and insomnia, add:

Rhizoma Anemarrhenae (*Zhi Mu*)
Semen Zizyphi Spinosae (*Zao Ren*)

Climacteric syndrome may be due to a vacuity of the *ren mai* and weakness of the *chong mai*. This gives rise to a vacuity of liver and kidney yin, an ascending hyperactivity of liver yang, or, in the extreme, a simultaneous weakness of kidney yang giving shape to a simultaneous vacuity of yin and yang with an upward attack of vacuity yang. This syndrome is appropriately treated with ***Er Xian Tang*** with modifications:

Herba Epimedii (*Xian Ling Pi*) 15g
Rhizoma Curculiginis Orchoidis (*Xian Mao*) 10g
Radix Morindae (*Ba Ji Tian*) 15g
Rhizoma Anemarrhenae (*Zhi Mu*) 10g, saltwater-fried
Cortex Phellodendri (*Huang Bai*) 10g, saltwater-fried
Radix Angelicae Sinensis (*Dang Gui*) 10g
Radix Lithospermi Seu Arnebiae (*Zi Cao*) 10g
Ramulus Uncariae Cum Uncis (*Gou Teng*) 15g, add last
Rhizoma Ligustici Wallichii (*Chuan Xiong*) 10g
raw Os Draconis (*Sheng Long Gu*) 15g
raw Concha Ostrea (*Sheng Mu Li*) 15g

In treating hypertension, regardless of the stage of the disease, one must level the liver and restrain the yang, taking care to nourish the heart and calm the spirit. In the case of recalcitrant hypertension, the treatment principles of disinhibiting dampness and vitalizing the blood, enriching and nourishing the heart and kidneys are primary and, when employed according to symptomology, will ameliorate the symptoms and markedly lower the blood pressure.

Wu Song-kang [I]

In my clinical treatment of hypertension, I divide this illness into syndromes of vacuity of liver and kidney yin with hyperactive liver yang, heart yin vacuity and hyperactivity of heart yang, simultaneous vacuity of kidney yin and yang, simultaneous vacuity of heart yin and yang, and endogenous wind. Hypertensive patterns of yin vacuity with hyperactivity of yang and a simultaneous vacuity of yin and yang all give rise to endogenous wind. There will be such symptoms as numbness of the extremities and face or the lips and tongue, involuntary spasms of the muscles and sinews, tremors of the hands and feet, and, in the extreme case, there will be wry mouth or the development of wind strike. The mechanisms of primary importance which engender endogenous wind are yin vacuity and hyperactivity of yang with a mutual flaring of wind and fire, a joint vacuity of qi and yin with a loss of nourishment of the sinew vessels creating a stasis of qi and blood. Clinically, ***Xi Feng Tang*** achieves a good result. The ingredients are:

Lumbricus (*Di Long*)
Rhizoma Ligustici Wallichii (*Chuan Xiong*)
Bombyx Batryticatus (*Jiang Can*)
Flos Immaturus Sophorae Japonicae (*Huai Hua Mi*)
Fructus Tribuli Terrestris (*Bai Ji Li*)

Based on variances in the pathomechanism, it is commonly combined with the following:

For liver and kidney yin vacuity with a mutual flaring of wind/fire, add:

Fructus Gardeniae Jasminoidis (*Zhi Zi*)
Cortex Radicis Moutan (*Dan Pi*)
Radix Ledeboureillae Sesloidis (*Fang Feng*)

Ramulus Mori Albi (*Sang Zhi*)
Er Zhi Wan [Composed of Fructus Ligustri Lucidi (*Nu Zhen Zi*) & Herba Ecliptae Prostratae (*Han Lian Cao*)]

For stasis in the channels and connecting vessels and blood not circulating smoothly, add:

Radix Astragali Seu Hedysari (*Huang Qi*)
Radix Angelicae Sinensis (*Dang Gui*)
Semen Pruni Persicae (*Tao Ren*)
Flos Carthami Tinctorii (*Hong Hua*)
Radix Psuedoginseng (*San Qi*)

For an accumulation of phlegm dampness in the connecting vessels, combine ***Xi Feng Tang*** and ***Huang Lian Wen Dan Tang***. For vacuity of yang with symptoms of chest *bi*, combine [the base prescription] with ***Zhi Shi Jiu Bai Gui Zhi Tang***. For women with a loss of regulation in the *chong* and *ren* giving rise to hypertension, combine [the base prescription] with ***Er Xian Tang***. Aside from these modifications, when one uses ***Xi Feng Tang***, the following additions are commonly made to effect a marked drop in blood pressure:

Semen Celosiae Argenteae (*Qing Xiang Zi*) 30g
Thallus Algae (*Kun Bu*) 20g

Case

A 54 year old male accountant had suffered from hypertension for many years and in the last month began suffering form daily bouts of dizziness, numbness of the upper extremities, lips, tongue, and facial area. He had difficulty walking and a wiry pulse. His tongue was red and was slightly greasy at the root and his blood pressure was 180/108. This all fell within the category of vacuity of liver and kidney yin and an internal movement of wind/yang. Appropriate treatment measures were to level the liver and extinguish wind and five doses of the following prescription were administered.

baked Lumbricus (*Di Long*) 12g
Flos Immaturus Sophorae Japonicae (*Huai Mi Hua*) 20g
Rhizoma Ligustici Wallichii (*Chuan Xiong*) 10g
Fructus Tribuli Terrestris (*Bai Ji Li*) 10g
charred Fructus Gardeniae Jasminoidis (*Zhi Zi*) 9g
Ramulus Uncariae Cum Uncis (*Gou Teng*) 9g
Cortex Radicis Moutan (*Dan Pi*) 9g
Semen Celosiae Argenteae (*Qing Xiang Zi*) 30g
Thallus Algae (*Kun Bu*) 20g

On a return visit there was a marked improvement in the numbness in the extremities, the dizziness was also diminished, and the blood pressure had decreased to 140/90. The patient continued on this basic prescription for more than 20 *ji*, his symptoms were completely cured, and his hypertension normalized.

Case

A 58 year old female cadre had suffered from hypertension for more than 10 years with symptoms of muddle-headedness and numbness of the upper extremities, particularly at the tips of the fingers. She had a tendency to intermittent tremors on the left side of her face, spiritual fatigue and weakness, a fine, wiry pulse and thin, white tongue fur. Her blood pressure was 200/108. All this fell into the category of dual weakness of the yin and qi with stasis of the vessels and connecting vessels. Appropriate treatment measures were to benefit the qi and quicken the blood, circulate the stasis, and penetrate the connecting vessels, and 5 doses of the following prescription were administered:

baked Lumbricus (*Di Long*) 12g
Rhizoma Ligustici Wallichii (*Chuan Xiong*) 10g
Bombyx Batryticatus (*Jiang Can*) 10g
Flos Immaturus Sophorae Japonicae (*Huai Mi Hua*) 30g
Fructus Tribuli Terrestris (*Bai Ji Li*) 20g
Semen Celoseae Argenteae (*Qing Xiang Zi*) 30g
Thallus Algae (*Kun Bu*) 30g
Radix Astragali Seu Hedysari (*Huang Qi*) 30g
Semen Pruni Persicae (*Tao Ren*) 10g
Flos Carthami Tinctorii (*Hong Hua*) 9g
Rhizoma Polygonati (*Huang Jing*) 10g
Radix Pseudoginseng (*San Qi*) 3g

Following this, the numbness of the extremities and facial tremors were markedly improved and the blood pressure decreased to 160/100. Subsequently, seven more doses of the base prescription were administered with the deletion of Rhizoma Polygonati and the addition of Rhizoma Gastrodiae Elatae (*Tian Ma*) 9g. The symptoms of internal wind were completely dispersed and the blood pressure remained at around 160/100. ***Xi Feng Tang*** with the following additions was administered, the symptoms stabilized, and the blood pressure was reduced to close to normal:

Semen Celosiae Argenteae (*Qing Xiang Zi*)
Thallus Algae (*Kun Bu*)
Fructus Aristolochiae (*Ma Dou Ling*)
Ramus Loranthi Seu Visci (*Sang Ji Sheng*)
Semen Pruni Persicae (*Tao Ren*)
Flos Carthami Tinctorii (*Hong Hua*)

Zhu Gu-ting [I]

In my treatment of hypertension, I find that differentiation based on the tongue is of primary importance. For instance, if the tongue body is red, then this is indicative of vacuity of yin and hyperactivity of yang. ***Qi Ju Di Huang Wan*** is indicated with the additions of agents to level the liver and restrain the yang, such as:

Ramulus Uncariae Cum Uncis (*Gou Teng*)
Concha Haliotidis (*Shi Jue Ming*)
Radix Scrophulariae Ningpoensis (*Yuan Shen*)
Tuber Ophiopogonis Japonicae (*Mai Dong*)

In the case of vacuity of yang with an insubstantiality of intestinal fluids, frequent constipation, and dry stools, the medicinals:

Radix Coquitus Rehmanniae (*Shu Di*)
Radix Scrophulariae Ningpoensis (*Yuan Shen*)
Tuber Ophiopogonis Japonicae (*Mai Dong*)

Form the ingredients of ***Zeng Ye Tang*** and in most patients the stools will become smooth and moist, and the visual dizziness and distension will become harmonized. Because the stomach qi circulates downward, the blood pressure can also be induced to descend. The practice of moistening the stool is also a measure for lowering the blood pressure.

If the tongue fur is rough and there is also severe visual dizziness and distending pain, then this is due to an upward attack of liver and gallbladder qi/fire. The administration of ***Long Dan Xie Gan Tang*** is appropriate with the addition of medicinals such as the following to clear the liver:

Spica Prunellae Vulgaris (*Xia Gu Cao*)

Folium Mori Albi (*Sang Ye*)
Concha Haliotidis (*Shi Jue Ming*)
Flos Chrysanthemi Morifolii (*Ju Hua*)
Ramulus Uncariae Cum Uncis (*Gou Teng*)
Fructus Tribuli Terrestris (*Bai Ji Li*)

If the tongue moss is slimy, then there is internal accumulation of phlegm turbidity and ascending attack of liver yang. If the tongue moss is white, then it is appropriate to administer ***Hou Po Ban Ling Tang*** with the addition of medicinals such as the following to level the liver:

Ramulus Uncariae Cum Uncis (*Gou Teng*)
Flos Chrysanthemi Morifolii (*Ju Hua*)
Concha Haliotidis (*Shi Jue Ming*)

If the tongue moss is yellow, then it is appropriate to administer ***Wen Dan Tang*** with additions such as the following to level the liver:

Snow peas (*Dou Quan*)
Caulis Bambusae In Taeniis (*Zhu Ru*)
Herba Eupatorii Fortnuei (*Pei Lan*)
Rhizoma Pinelliae Ternatae (*Ban Xia*)
Sclerotium Poriae Cocoris (*Fu Ling*)
Ramulus Uncariae Cum Uncis (*Gou Teng*)
Flos Chrysanthemi Morifolii (*Ju Hua*)
Concha Haliotidis (*Shi Jue Ming*)

In the case of an elderly person with weakness of water and effulgence of wood causing an upward attack of wind/yang and symptoms of vertigo, then the administration of ***Liu Wei Di Huang Wan*** is appropriate with the addition of ingredients such as the following to clear the liver, restrain the yang, and extinguish wind:

Flos Chrysanthemi Morifolii (*Ju Hua*)
Concha Haliotidis (*Shi Jue Ming*)
Ramulus Uncariae Cum Uncis (*Gou Teng*)
Folium Mori Albi (*Sang Ye*)

Whenever I treat hypertension, I invariably use Flos Chrysanthemi Morifolii, Concha Haliotidis, and Ramulus Uncariae Cum Uncis and, based on the tongue fur and changes in the body, will make modifications accordingly.

Wei Zhang-chun [I]

Symptoms of tidal fever and drastic fluctuations in diastolic pressure are indicative of a surging ascension of liver fire. For this condition, ***Huang Qin Xie Huo Tang*** is prescribed which contains the following ingredients.

To clear the liver and drain heat:

Radix Scutellariae Baicalensis (*Huang Qin*)
Fructus Gardeniae Jasminoidis (*Zhi Zi*)
Rhizoma Coptidis Chinensis (*Huang Lian*)

To transform yin, soften the liver, and cool the blood, the addition of sweet and sour agents:

Radix Albus Paeoniae Lactiflorae (*Bai Shao*)
Radix Glycyrrhizae (*Gan Cao*)

To level the liver and extinguish wind:

Radix Uncariae Cum Uncis (*Gou Teng*)

To supplement the liver and kidneys and circulate the blood downward:

Radix Achyranthis Bidentatae (*Niu Xi*)

Longstanding illness with a constant elevation of both diastolic and systolic pressure is indicative of hyperactive ascension of liver yang. Therefore, it is appropriate to level the liver and descend counterflow. [For this,] he prescribed a medication of his own formulation ***Jiang Ya Tiao Gan Tang*** containing the following ingredients.

To cool the liver and course wind and clear head wind:

Scapus Eriocaulonis (*Gu Jing Cao*)
Spica Prunellae Vulgaris (*Xia Gu Cao*)
Flos Chrysanthemi Indici (*Ye Ju Hua*)

To level the liver and extinguish wind:

Ramulus Uncariae Cum Uncis (*Gou Teng*)

To soften the liver and lower blood pressure:

Semen Cassiae Torae (*Jue Ming Zi*)

To fortify the liver and kidneys while simultaneously promoting the circulation of blood downward:

Herba Ecliptae Prostratae (*Han Lian Cao*)
Ramus Loranthi Seu Visci (*Sang Ji Sheng*)
Radix Achyranthis Bidentatae (*Niu Xi*)

Symptoms of heavy headedness while the legs are light and especially high diastolic blood pressure are indicative of repletion above and vacuity below. For this condition, he prescribes a medication of his own formulation, ***Qi Ju Di Huang Tang,*** which contains the following ingredients.

To supplement vacuity and bank up the root, fill in the essence and enrich the kidneys:

Fructus Lycii Chinensis (*Gou Qi*)
Radix Coquitus Rehmanniae (*Shu Di*)
Fructus Corni Officinalis (*Shan Zhu Yu*)
Herba Ecliptae Prostratae (*Han Lian Cao*)

To nourish the liver and disperse wind, clear above:

Flos Chrysanthemi Morifolii (*Ju Hua*)

To clear the liver and lower blood pressure:

Semen Cassiae Torae (*Jue Ming Zi*)
Ramulus Uncariae Cum Uncis (*Gou Teng*)

To moisten the yin portion and drain vacuity fire:

Rhizoma Alismatis (*Ze Xie*)

To cool the liver, disperse wind, and penetrate the connecting vessels:

Ramulus Mori Albi (*Sang Zhi*)

To promote the downward circulation of stagnant heat:

Radix Achyranthis Bidentatae (*Niu Xi*)

Chen Ze-lin [I]

The addition of 3-4 medicinals which are specifically antihypertensive [to a given prescription] will enhance antihypertensive effect as well as the amelioration of symptoms. Nevertheless, pattern discrimination (*bian zheng*) must be combined with disease discrimination (*bian bing*) in order to achieve an optimal result using Chinese medicine. Our forbearer, Chen Yao-tang, a practitioner of old Chinese medicine, did not eschew the use of Radix Praeparatus Aconiti Carmichaeli (*Fu Zi*) and Cortex Cinnamomi [in the treatment of hypertension] recognizing that if the discrimination of syndromes was correct, then bold measures could be appropriate. Nonetheless, the dosages should be small and combined with medicinals such as Radix Rehmanniae and Concha Haliotidis. For those not willing to take Chinese herbs long term, our forbearers prescribed a powder of Radix Puerariae Lobatae as a beverage. Others used a packaged Chrysanthemum tea as a typical drink to lower blood pressure. Still others used sliced Radix Polygoni Multiflori as a prophylactic against angiosclerosis. In assessing the risk for wind strike, if clotting factors are excessively high, then I advocate the use of medicinals to quicken the blood, transform stasis, and protect against excessive clotting, such as the following:

Radix Salviae Miltorrhizae (*Dan Shen*)
Radix Rubrus Paeoniae Lactiflorae (*Chi Shao*)
Flos Chrysanthemi Morifolii (*Ju Hua*)
Lignum Aquilariae Agallochae (*Chen Xiang*)
Semen Pruni Persicae (*Tao Ren*)

In the case of ischemic stroke where there is a tendency towards accumulation of thrombocytes, stroke resulting from an overflow of blood into the brain, this is a condition which cannot be easily predicted.

Case Histories

1. Zhu Xi-qi [IV]

Patient Gui, a 57 year old male.

His initial visit was on December 9th, 1963. [The patient reported that] his blood pressure was 230/130 millimeters of mercury. He had been hypertensive for many years and had a rash and impatient nature. This morning, his tongue had become rigid and he suffered from numbness in his fingers, mental dizziness, flowery vision, and an unstable gait. His face was cinnabar red and his tongue was deviated to the side. His mouth [and breath] were foul and offensive. His pulse was wiry and rapid and his tongue had a thin, yellow coat. [The diagnosis was] ascending attack of liver yang, downward drawing of kidney yin [*xia ji shen yin*], accumulation of heat in the *yang ming*. The treatment plan was to drain heat and unblock the bowels, drain the liver and restrain the yang.

powdered Cornu Antelopis (*Ling Yang Jiao*) swallowed separately, 0.6g
Ramulus Uncariae Cum Uncis (*Gou Teng*) 12g, added at the end
Radix Gentianae Scabrae (*Long Dan Cao*) 6g
raw Radix Et Rhizoma Rhei (*Da Huang*) 6g, added at the end
Spica Prunellae Vulgaris (*Xia Gu Cao*) 12g
Flos Chrysanthemi Indici (*Ye Ju Hua*) 12g
Semen Cassiae Torae (*Jue Ming Zi*) 30g
Radix Scutellariae Baicalensis (*Huang Qin*) 6g
Concha Haliotidis (*Shi Jue Ming*) 30g, precooked
Margarita (*Zhen Zhu*) 30g, precooked

2 *ji*[1]

The second visit was on December 11th. [The patient's] blood pressure was 180/110 millimeters of mercury. His blood pressure had dropped after taking the medicine and his bowels had moved. Nonetheless, he had a headache, flowery vision, and facial redness due to ascending fire. He was loquacious and jovial, drool flowed from the corners of his mouth, his left hand was numb, and he swayed when he walked. His pulse was thin and wiry and his tongue had a thin, yellow coat. The ascending attack of liver yang had not been extinguished and again measures were employed to drain the liver and drain heat, assisted by measures for restraining the yang.

powdered Cornu Antelopis (*Ling Yang Jiao*) swallowed separately, 0.6g
Concha Haliotidis (*Shi Jue Ming*) 30g, precooked
Margarita (*Zhen Zhu*) 30g, precooked
Radix Gentianae Scabrae (*Long Dan Cao*) 6g
Cortex Radicis Moutan (*Dan Pi*) 9g
Spica Prunellae Vulgaris (*Xia Gu Cao*) 12g
Herbae Siegesbeckiae(*Xi Jian Cao*) 15g
Semen Firmianae (*Wu Tong Zi*) 30g
Radix Salviae Miltorrhizae (*Dan Shen*) 9g
Radix Scutellariae Baicalensis (*Huang Qin*) 9g
Semen Cassiae Torae (*Jue Ming Zi*) 30g
Semen Leonuri Heterphylli (*Chong Wei Zi*) 12g

2 *ji*

---

1 The word *ji* literally means formula. It cannot be translated accurately as either dose, packet, day's supply, or any other term. Since translating it literally as formula seems awkward in English, we have chosen to leave it in Chinese *pinyin*.

The third visit was on December 14th. [The patient's] blood pressure was 150/90 millimeters of mercury. His blood pressure was consistently lower, his tongue was no longer deviated, and his headache had diminished. He was loquacious, jovial, and animated. There was a great deal of phlegm in his throat, his speech was inhibited, and he drooled. His pulse was wiry and thin and he had a thin coat on his tongue. The wind/fire was gradually being extinguished. However phlegm turbidity had attached itself internally. Although he was out of danger, caution was necessary to guard against the perils lying ahead. [The treatment measures were to] balance the liver and extinguish wind, transform phlegm and clear heat.

Herba Siegesbeckiae (*Xi Jian Cao*) 12g
Semen Cassiae Torae (*Jue Ming Zi*) 30g
Spica Prunellae Vulgaris (*Xia Ku Cao*) 12g
Radix Salviae Miltorrhizae (*Dan Shen*) 9g
Rhizoma Pinelliae Ternatae (*Ban Xia*) 6g
Rhizoma Curcumae (*Jiang Huang*) 9g
Rhizoma Arisaematis (*Nan Xing*) 6g
Concretio Siliceae Bambusae (*Tian Zhu Huang*) 6g
Cortex Radicis Moutan (*Dan Pi*) 9g
Bombyx Batryticatus (*Jiang Can*) 9g
Concha Haliotidis (*Shi Jue Ming*) 30g, precooked
Margarita (*Zhen Zhu*) 30g, precooked

4 *ji*

The fourth visit was on December 12th. [The patient's] blood pressure was 160\100 millimeters of mercury. His loquacious and jovial nature had overall changed somewhat for the better. He remained rash and impatient as before, with mental dizziness, poor sleep, and ascension of fire into the head and face. [The diagnosis was that of] exuberance of heart fire with a tendency to effulgence of liver yang. Therefore, [treatment measures were] to clear the heart and descend fire, balance the liver and restrain the yang.

Herba Siegesbeckiae (*Xi Jian Cao*) 12g
Rhizoma Coptidis Chinensis (*Huang Lian*) 3g
burnt Fructus Gardeniae Jasminoidis (*Zhi Zi*) 9g
Embryon Forsythiae (*Lian Qiao Xin*) 12g
Concha Haliotidis (*Shi Jue Ming*) 12g, precooked
Margarita (*Zhen Zhu*) 30g, precooked
Plastrum Testudinis (*Gui Ban*) 12g, precooked
Concha Ostreae (*Mu Li*) 30g, precooked
Ramulus Uncariae Cum Uncis (*Gou Teng*) 12g, added at the end
Fructus Tribuli Terrestris (*Bai Ji Li*) 12g
Radix Salviae Miltiorrhizae (*Dan Shen*) 9g
raw Radix Albus Paeoniae Lactiflorae (*Bai Shao*) 9g
Magnetitum (*Ci Shi*) 30g, precooked

5 *ji*

The fifth visit was on December 19, 1964. [The patient's] blood pressure was 150/96 millimeters of mercury. The cardiac vexation had cleared up, the palpitations had largely diminished, and the ascension of fire had been constrained as well. Again the plan was to balance the liver and restrain the yang, nourish the blood and calm the spirit.

Radix Salviae Miltiorrhizae (*Dan Shen*) 9g
Caulis Polygoni Multiflori (*Ye Jiao Teng*) 30g
Fructus Tribuli Terrestris (*Bai Ji Li*) 9g
Semen Zizyphi Spinosae (*Zao Ren*) 9g
Flos Immaturus Sophorae Japonicae (*Huai Mi Hua*) 12g
Magnetitum (*Ci Shi*) 30g, precooked
Concha Ostreae (*Mu Li*) 30g, precooked
husked Sorghum (*Bei Shu Mi*) 12g
Spica Prunellae Vulgaris (*Xia Ku Cao*) 9g

Cortex Albizziae (*He Huan Pi*) 12g

5 *ji*

Comment: The evolution of this case is related mainly to the emotions. The immediate cause was anger which had caused the qi to ascend. This caused liver yang to shoot up, binding dryness of the bowels, upward purgation of accumulated heat within the *yang ming*, congestion phlegm heat, and ascension of qi fire. The wind rode on the strength of the fire, and fire depended upon the power of the wind such that it manifested with the immediate force of a prairie fire. Thus, the sudden development of lingual rigidity and inhibition, headache, numbness in the fingers, and unclear speech were considered an acute development. Since it was acute, the branch was treated with powdered Cornu Antelopi to balance the liver and extinguish the wind. This was assisted by Radix Gentianae Scabrae, Concha Haliotidis, Radix Scutellariae Baicalensis, and Spica Prunellae Vulgaris which are bitter, cold, and drain the upward exuberance of fire. Concha Haliotidis and Margarita balance the liver and restrain the yang. Flos Chrysanthemi Indici and Ramulus Uncariae Cum Uncis clear the ascension of yang. Cortex Radicis Moutan cools the blood and Radix Et Rhizoma Rhei quickly purges the *yang ming* bowels. When the bowels are unblocked, the qi/fire will follow suit. The wind is leveled and the heat drained. Thus the firewood is removed from beneath the cauldron.

This illness is primarily due to an effulgence of wood with flaring of fire generating wind, an upward counterflow of qi and blood, and sudden congestion of phlegm drool. The *Su Wen* states: "Major inversion [is due to] a joint ascension of qi and blood." As soon as the flaring of qi has been balanced and extinguished, treatment is aimed at the root. Although the phlegm turbidity is the main focus in this illness, if the vacuity is given consideration, then enrichment and fortification are indicated. Enriching medicinals, however, tend to be greasy and are all contraindicated with phlegm turbidity. Therefore, restraining the yang and settling counterflow via medicinals predominantly in the shell category is the primary focus. This is because their salty, cold, and heavy nature is capable of sinking and downbearing and so stabilizes the striving ascendency of qi/fire. The qi and taste of all [these medicinals] is light and so does not [further] obstruct the phlegm turbidity. The prescription, therefore, contains Concha Haliotidis, Margarita, and Concha Ostreae to restrain the yang and settle counterflow, level the wind and downbear fire. Nourishment of water and the moistening of wood, support of yin and restraint of yang are the major measures needed in order to achieve a result in treatment.

2. Gong Wen-de

Critical hypertension

Critical hypertension implies an acutely elevated blood pressure. This is simultaneously accompanied by the essential clinical expressions of headache, mental dizziness, palpitations, nausea, obstructed vision, and, ultimately, stupor and convulsive spasm. According to Chinese medical pattern differentiation, a "violent exuberance of liver fire" or "depletion of true yin with ascending attack of wind/yang" are the most commonly seen patterns. Nevertheless, there are yin patterns which are similar to yang [patterns], and these conditions are both ominous and dangerous. In the medical discussions of the old masters, [Zhang] Zhongjing's measures were employed for this illness with the use of ***Bai Tong Tang*** with additions.

Zhang Feng-jiao's Prescription

Composition:

blast-fried pieces of Radix Praeparatus Aconiti Carmichaeli (*Fu Zi*) 9-12g (precooked)
Rhizoma Desiccata Zingiberis (*Gan Jiang*) 4.5g
Bulbus Allii Fistulosi (*Cong Bai*) 4 pieces
calcined Os Draconis (*Long Gu*) 30g
calcined Concha Ostreae (*Mu Li*) 30g
baked Fructus Schizandrae Chinensis (*Wu Wei*) 3g

Explanation of the prescription:

This prescription is ***Bai Tong Tang*** with additions. It is also known as ***Bai Tong Lian Yang Tang.*** Radix Praeparatus Aconiti Carmichaeli and Rhizoma Desiccata Zingeberis in this prescription defeat the yin and return the yang. Bulbus Allii Fistulosi perfuses and unblocks the repelled yang both above and below. The addition of Os Draconis, Concha Ostreae, and Fructus Schizandrae Chinensis constrains the yang and guards against desertion. The combination of all these medicinals is effective in rapidly returning the yang and stemming counterflow.

Appropriate Pattern: Critical hypertension within a pattern pertaining to heart and kidney yang depletion and yin exuberance repelling yang

Modification Measures:

1. [For symptoms of] counterflow chill in the four extremities and loss of consciousness with a slight pulse on the verge of expiration, all pertaining to a depletion heart and kidney yang causing a violent desertion of force, add red Radix Panacis Ginseng 9g (decocted separately in soluble preparation), Herba Cistanchis

(*Rou Cong Rong*) 12g, and Radix Morindae 12g for superlative supplementation the true yang and to guard against sudden desertion.

2. [For symptoms of] dripping perspiration, extreme depletion of the qi fluids, and concern that the yang will subjugate the yin and transform it, add Herba Dendrobii (*Shi Hu*) 12g and Tuber Ophiopogonis Japonicae 12g, to enrich the yin and harmonize the yang and to guard against the separation of yin and yang.

3. [For symptoms of] obvious facial redness, tidal fever, and unresolved vexation agitation, add Depositum Urinae Praeparatum (*Ren Zhong Bai*) (in the place of human urine) with the implication that the yin leads the yang and this assists in the descent and restraint of the floating yang.

4. If the hands grasp at emptiness, there is a forceful stirring of wind and spasmodic inversion. Therefore, add Rhizoma Gastrodiae Elatae 9g and Ramulus Uncariae Cum Uncis 12g (added last).

Case history

Liu, a 48 year old male, was diagnosed on November 22, 1962. He had suffered from hypertension for more than a decade and, in the past two days, had experienced intense mental dizziness which was particularly intense. [There was] photophobia, unclear vision, a red face, palpitations, and occasional vexation. [His] body was cold and he preferred to be recumbent. There was a dripping, cool sweat, lack of warmth in the four extremities, a deep, fine, and slight pulse. His tongue was pale, plump, and tender. His blood pressure was 200/120 millimeters of mercury. This pattern pertained to a depletion of heart and kidney yang and an ascension of repelled yang. The state of his illness was critical and I was alert to prevent any sudden changes in his condition as there was concern that it might transform into an inversion desertion pattern. The plan was to defeat the yin and return the yang, perfuse and unblock both above and below. An imitation of the *Shang Han Lun's* ***Bai Tong Tang*** with additions was administered to aggressively shift this dynamic. The prescription consisted of:

blast-fried pieces of Radix Praeparatus Aconiti Carmichaeli (*Fu Zi*) 9g, precooked
Rhizoma Desiccata Zingeberis (*Gan Jiang*) 4.5g
Bulbus Allii Fistulosi (*Cong Bai*) 4 pieces
calcined Os Draconis (*Long Gu*) 30g
calcined Concha Ostreae (*Mu Li*) 30g
baked Fructus Schizandrae Chinensis (*Wu Wei*) 3g
Depositum Urinae Preparatum (*Ren Zhong Bai*) 30g

1 *ji*

After administration of 1 dose of the above prescription, the mental dizziness and palpitations clearly diminished, the facial redness disappeared, the extremities warmed up, and the pulse shifted and recovered its strength. With continued administration of another dose, the condition stabilized and his blood pressure was 160/100 millimeters of mercury.

3. Yan Cang-shan [IV]

Patient Yang, a 44 year old female

Initial visit: [The patient suffered from] hypertension, thoracic oppression, and upflow nausea with extreme mental dizziness and pain. [She also had a] slippery, wiry pulse and a thin, slimy tongue coat, all of which were indicative of wind in the *jue yin* sending ministerial fire [upward]. There was a mutual fanning of wind and fire scurrying up the mountain [vertex] which resulted in dizziness and pain. At the same time, there was a loss of harmonious downbearing within the stomach resulting in thoracic oppression and upflow nausea. This was not a mild condition (the blood pressure was 230/135 millimeters mercury) and it was imperative to prevent any sudden negative changes. [The plan] was to urgently balance the liver and restrain the yang, harmonize the stomach, and downbear counterflow. Observation of some relaxation in the force [of the counterflow] would be a good sign.

Carapax Eretmochelyos (*Dai Mao*) 6g, pre-cooked
ginger-prepared Rhizoma Pinelliae Ternatae (*Ban Xia*) 9g
raw Concha Haliotidis (*Shi Jue Ming*) 15g, pre-cooked
Flos Chrysanthemi Morifolii (*Ju Hua*) 6g
carbonized Herba Menthae (*Bo He*) 3g, added last
baked Bombyx Batryticatus (*Jiang Can*) 9g
Caulis Bambusae In Taeniis (*Zhu Ru*) 6g
ginger-prepared Rhizoma Coptidis Chinensis (*Huang Lian*) 2.4g
Ramulus Uncariae Cum Uncis (*Gou Teng*) 9g, added last
Niu Huang Qing Xin Wan, 1 pill, dissolved in liquid and taken orally

Second visit: The patient suffered from mental dizziness and pain, torpid intake and upflow nausea, palpitations, and shortness of breath. Her tongue coat was thin, yellow, and slimy and her pulse was deep and a little slippery. The conflict in the symptoms was due to a loss of transportation within spleen/earth which was generating phlcgm. Since the phlegm generated heat and the heat generated wind, the blood pressure became excessively elevated, and there was a hyperactive counterflow of wind/yang. The plan was to transform phlegm turbidity, harmonize the stomach, and balance the liver rather than placing a great deal of weight on draining the liver.

Radix Glehniae Littoralis (*Sha Shen*) 9g
Caulis Bambusae In Taeniis (*Zhu Ru*) 6 g
Succus Bambusae-prepared Rhizoma Pinelliae Ternatae (*Ban Xia*) 9g
Pericarpium Citri Reticulatae (*Chen Pi*) 6g
Fructus Tribuli Terrestris (*Bai Ji Li*) 9g
husked Sorghum (*Bei Shu Mi*) 9g, wrapped
Testa Glycines (*Dou Yi*) 9g
fried Fructus Citri Seu Ponciri (*Zhi Qiao*) 4.5g
Flos Chrysanthemi Morifolii (*Ju Hua*) 56g
raw Concha Haliotidis (*Shi Jue Ming*) 15g, pre-cooked
Sclerotium Poriae Cocoris (*Fu Ling*) 9g
raw Semen Coicis Lachryma-jobi (*Yi Yi Ren*) 9g
Ramulus Uncariae Cum Uncis (*Gou Teng*) 9g, added last

Third visit: Using measures for harmonizing the stomach, balancing the liver, and transforming turbidity, the *pi* oppression in the middle warmer was immediately soothed and the pulse picture improved as well. The mental dizziness and pain gradually diminished, the torpid intake gradually improved, and the upflow nausea also ceased. The slimy tongue coat, however, had still not entirely been transformed, so changes in dosage were made to the original prescription.

Radix Glehniae Littoralis (*Sha Shen*) 9g
raw Concha Haliotidis (*Shi Jue Ming*) 15g, pre-cooked
Caulis Bambusae In Taeniis (*Zhu Ru*) 6g
fried Pericarpium Citri Reticulatae (*Chen Pi*) 4.5g
Fructus Citri Seu Ponciri (*Zhi Qiao*) 4.5g
fried Fructus Immaturus Citri Seu Ponciri (*Zhi Shi*) 6g
Herba Eupatorii Fortunei (*Pei Lan*) 6g
raw Semen Coicis Lachryma-jobi (*Yi Yi Ren*) 9g
Fructus Tribuli Terrestris (*Bai Ji Li*) 9g
husked Sorghum (*Bei Shu Mi*) 6g, wrapped
Fructus Germinatus hordei Vulgaris (*Mai Ya*) 12g

Fructus Germinatus Oryzae Sativae (*Gu Ya*) 12g
Sclerotium Poriae Cocoris (*Fu Ling*) 9g

Commentary: The intense headache and the contraction of the flesh on the face at the corners of the mouth were grave symptoms of ascending counterflow of wind/yang and a precursor to wind strike. Nevertheless, the inclusion of liver-balancing and yang-restraining [medicinals] yielded no obvious effect. This was chiefly because the pulse did not match the pattern and on the contrary was deep and slightly slippery. This was due to loss of healthy transportation within the spleen, an accumulation of dampness generating phlegm, and wind/yang coercing an upward counterflow of phlegm turbidity with symptoms of thoracic oppression and slimy tongue coat. The transformation of phlegm was, therefore, primarily assisted by measures for balancing the liver. If the stomach and spleen are transporting, then phlegm is not generated, the root is corrected, the source is cleared, and the pulse pattern is in agreement [with the symptoms]. Thus, with the appropriate handiwork, there is a cure.

STICKS AND STONES

The Chinese Medical Treatment of Bone Fractures

Introduction

Acupuncturists and herbalists in the United States are not often called upon to set broken bones since this is generally outside the scope of their expertise. It is not uncommon, however, for practitioners to find themselves placed in the position of facilitating a more rapid recovery from a traumatic incident once the bone has been set. In this situation, acupuncture is an obvious therapeutic choice. However, despite the usefulness of distal points, acupuncture can leave something to be desired when confronted with a carapace of fiberglass or plaster[1]. The realm of traditional Chinese medical orthopedics encompasses bone setting techniques, manual manipulation, physical therapy, and medical gymnastics such as *dao yin* and *qi gong*, as well as acupuncture and herbal medicine. While it is unusual for an individual to have a true expertise in every facet of this specialty, acupuncture and herbal medicine applied in conjunction with skilled manual therapies is both practical and remarkably effective.

---

1 This points up an one obvious difference in the way fractures are treated here and in Asia. They more often end up in a cast in the west, leaving potentially useful topical and local therapies to the time when the cast is removed. It is pleasing to note however, that there is a trend toward both mobilizing fractures and removing casts earlier and earlier in the course of western orthopedic therapies.

The Shi family of Shanghai, PRC are among the most renowned orthopedic specialists in the field of Chinese medicine. The following article by Shi Yang-shan, the son of grand master Shi Xiao-shan outlines the basic tenants of Chinese medical orthopedics as practiced by his family. His discussions on manipulative techniques should be of clinical interest to those specifically trained in manipulation. Those not trained in this area will find it a concise overview of Chinese orthopedic modalities. The prescriptions will be of use to any herbal practitioner who has ever confronted a bone fracture. Shi Yang-shan's article is followed by an essay by Shi Wei-zhi which is primarily herbal in nature, and which emphasizes specific formulae and medicinals based on the location of the injury.

Theoretical Discussions

Shi Yang-shan [I]

Traumatology and the treatment of bone fractures as it is practiced by the Shi family emphasizes the entire conceptual framework of the medical system of our homeland. It stresses the discrimination of syndromes in both internal and external treatment. The healing of fractures and the speedy recovery of bodily function can only be achieved by recognizing the value of the organic coordination of manual reduction techniques, stabilization, internal administration, and topical application of medicinals, along with the integration of both movement and quietude. In diagnosis and treatment, attention must be paid to the following aspects.

1. The employment of hand techniques which are both firm and gentle are most preferable. When executing manual techniques, one should, as far as possible, achieve a satisfactory and complete reduction on the first attempt. This should be done with a

manual technique which is both firm and gentle so as to avoid further injury to tendons and bones which have already been damaged or broken. For instance, the reduction of a bone fracture at a joint cannot be overly violent. When applying traction, it should be vigorous and steady, with the exertion evenly distributed and maintained continuously. The physical contact should be such that the force is mediated internally. Rotation should be applied with a light touch. [Using this approach], a severely rotated fracture within a joint will often recover fully.

2. External fixation [*i.e.*, splinting/casting,etc.] is characterized by stabilization and regularization. Unstabilized bone fractures commonly employ a multileveled stabilization technique which is safe and secure. The innermost strata of regularization consists of the topical application of medicinals using a degreased cotton cloth, evenly distributed around the area. Pieces of China fir (木杉) may be used as is necessary, tailored into different shapes, on top of which is applied a pressure cushion. This will enable the broken ends to knit properly. Finally a bandage is employed and wrapped around the dressing to secure it. For the outer layer, a cylindrical cardboard splint or a hard wood splint is used, wrapped in a bandage to secure it. For joints or internal fractures of the joints, the stabilization must extend beyond the joint itself and, if necessary, when applying traction.

3. Appropriate use of medicinals, both administered internally and applied topically, is indicated. The application of topical medicinals should be at the site of the fracture. Of significant value in the recovery of bone fractures is application of such

proven prescriptions as ***San Se Fu Yao***[2], to rid swelling and arrest pain, ***San Huang Gao***[3] to clear heat, cool the blood and rid stasis, ***Hong Yu Gao***[4] to protect the skin and flesh, and ***Xu Gu Gao***[5] to promote the healing of the bone fracture. In the latter stages use ***Shang Gao Yao***[6] to warm the channels, quicken the blood, and arrest pain. The vigorous adhesive capacity of these plasters actually enhances the functions of stability overall.

4. The internal administration of medicinals should treat the entire [clinical picture] according to a discrimination of syndromes, so as to speed up the assimilation of blood stasis,

---

2 *San Se Fu Yao* ingredients are: Semen Vitex (*Man Jing Zi*) 8 parts, Cortex Pternopetali (*Zi Jin Sha*) fried black 8 parts, Fructus Chaenomelis (*Mu Gua*) 2 parts, Radix Salvia Miltiorrhizae (*Dan Shen*) 2 parts, Radix Notopterygii (*Qiang Huo*) 2 parts, Radix Paeoniae Rubrae (*Chi Shao*) 2 parts, Radix Angelica Dahuricae (*Bai Zhi*) 2 parts, Rhizoma Curcumae (*Yu Jin*) 2 parts, Radix Angelicae Duhuo (*Du Huo*) 2 parts, Radix Glycyrrhizae (*Gan Cao*), 1/2 part, Radix Gentianae Macrophyllae (*Qin Jiao*) 1 part, Radix Trichosanthes (*Tian Huo Fen*) 2 parts, Radix Achyranthes (*Niu Xi*) 2 parts, Radix Ligusticii Wallichii (*Chuan Xiong*) 1 part, Fructus Forsythiae (*Lian Qiao*) 1 part, Radix Clematidis (*Wei Ling Xian*) 2 parts, Radix Cocculi (*Mu Fang Ji*) 2 parts, Radix Ledebouriellae (*Fang Feng*) 2 parts, Semen Strychnos (*Ma Qian Zi*) 2 parts

3 The ingredients of *San Huang Gao* are unavailable. There are, however, a variety of plasters which are readily available in the West which achieve similar ends. Many of the topical applications mentioned in this article are considered to be proprietary secrets by the hospitals in which they are used. Even in those cases where the ingredients are available, the method of formulation is often not cited. This is the case, for instance, in *San Se Fu Yao*.

4 *Hong Yu Gao*'s ingredients are unavailable.

5 *Xi Gu Dan*'s ingredients are unavailable.

6 *Shang Gao Yao*'s ingredients are unavailable.

disperse swelling and pain, and to completely heal the fracture. [These medicinals] are then gradually diminished as the symptoms disappear. This [detail] cannot be overlooked. My father, the late Shi Xiao-shan, a senior Chinese physician, drafted ***Xin Shang Xu Duan Tang*** and its effects for dispersing swelling, arresting pain, and binding the bones are considerable. In the latter stages of bone fractures ***Tiao Zhong Xu Gu Tang*** is typically used, [the ingredients of which are]:

Radix Astragali Seu Hedysari (*Huang Qi*) 15g
Radix Codonopsis Pilosulae (*Dang Shen*) 15g
Rhizoma Atractylodis Macrcocephalae (*Bai Zhu*) 15g
Radix Albus Paeoniae Lactiflorae (*Bai Shao*) 15g
Pericarpium Citri Reticulatae (*Chen Pi*) 5g
Radix Rehmanniae (*Sheng Di*) 15g
Radix Glycyrrhizae (*Gan Cao*) 3g
Radix Angelicae Sinensis (*Dang Gui*) 10g
Rhizoma Drynariae (*Gu Sui Bu*) 15g
Pyritum (*Zi Ran Tong*) 15g
Sclerotium Poriae Cocoris (*Fu Ling*) 15g
Gummum Olibani (*Ru Xiang*) 15g

Yi Yuan Xu Gu Tang may also be used to supplement the qi and blood, supplement the spleen and stomach, and benefit the liver and kidneys, as well as promoting rapid healing of the fracture, supplementing the sinews, and strengthening the bones. It is also remarkably effective in treating retarded healing of fractures. (The ingredients are:)

Radix Dioscoreae Oppositae (*Shan Yao*) 15g
Radix Coquitus Rehmanniae (*Shu Di*) 12g
Radix Dipsaci (*Xu Duan*) 10g
Radix Salviae Miltiorrhizae (*Dan Shen*) 10g
Cornu Cervi Degelatinum (*Lu Jiao Shuang*) 10g
Fructus Corni Officinalis (*Shan Zhu Yu*) 10g

Fructus Psoraleae Corylifoliae (*Bu Gu Zhi*) 10g
Plastrum Testudinis (*Gui Ban*) 12g
Sclerotium Poriae Cocoris (*Fu Ling*) 12g
Rhizoma Drynariae (*Gu Sui Bu*) 12g
Flos Carthami Tinctorii (*Hong Hua*) 3g
Caulis Milletiae Seu Spatholobi (*Ji Xue Teng*) 15g

In clinical practice, a patient's extremities may remain swollen and distended for years, even though the fracture has healed, and the splint has been removed. To these patients ***Shang Gao***[7] is applied topically and physical therapy urged. Internal application of ***Bu Yang Huan Wu Tang*** is indicated.

Rhizoma Atractylodis (*Cang Zhu*)
Sclerotium Poriae Cocoris (*Fu Ling*)
Rhizoma Alismatis (*Ze Xie*)
Ramulus Cinnamomi (*Gui Zhi*)

The following may be added to warm and transform phlegm stasis for a particularly good result:

Radix Aconiti (*Wu Tou*)
Rhizoma Arisaematis (*Nan Xing*)
Herba Euphorbiae Helioscopiae (*Ze Qi*)

In the case of a patient who suffers from weakness, soreness, and pain following a bone fracture with rigidity of the joints, or climatic changes affecting the joint and resulting in soreness and pain, all of these symptoms fall within the category of stasis following a fracture, soreness and pain following a bone fracture with rigidity of the joints, or climatic changes affecting the joint and resulting in soreness and pain. All of these symptoms fall

[7] *Shang Gao*'s ingredients are unavailable.

within the category of stasis following a fracture. In the case of an attack of wind cold damp pathogens such that the sinew, the vessels, qi and blood are not dredged and unfettered, measures are indicated to soothe the sinew and enliven the blood, [rid] obstruction and unfetter the collaterals. This should be combined with administration of fumigations, fomentations, acupuncture, and *dao yin* exercises to achieve the effect.

5. Equal attention should be paid to the sinew and bone and they should be treated together. This is because after a bone fracture there will certainly be an injury to the sinew as well. This is particularly true [when a fracture occurs] near a joint or within a joint itself. Often there is simultaneous tearing and injury of the soft tissue surrounding the joint. Clinically it often happens that the restoration of the sinew is slow compared to the mending of the bone fracture itself. Consequently, my late father, in promoting complete reduction and stabilization of bone fractures, simultaneously used manual manipulation of the sinew to facilitate recovery of the fascia as well. When changing the herbal dressing, he would from time to time rotate the joint, pressing and kneading the sinew and fascia in the area surrounding the injured joint, in an effort to achieve the goal of "truing the bones and making the sinew supple". Moreover the patient should be encouraged to move and exercise the joint. Consequently, the development of joint rigidity, fascial contracture, and other sequelae will be relatively minor.

Shi Wei-zhi [I]

In the treatment of closed bone fractures, except when employing manipulative techniques and applying topical medications, administration of internal therapy must be based on the differentiations of the three stages of bone fracture. The purpose of this is to promote growth and fusion of the severed bone, functionally speeding recovery. Yet one must discriminate between various locations since bone fractures to the extremities are different from those to the trunk. In the first stage of a bone fracture to the extremities with swelling, pain, distension, and soreness one typically uses:

Radix Angelicae Sinensis (*Dang Gui*) 10g
Radix Rubrus Paeoniae Lactiflorae (*Chi Shao*) 6g
Rhizoma Ligustici Wallichii (*Chuan Xiong*) 9g
Semen Pruni Persicae (*Tao Ren*) 9g
Lignum Sappanis (*Su Mu*) 9g·
Pyritum (*Zi Ran Tong*) 9g
Eupolyphagae Seu Opisthoplatiae (*Tu Bie Chong*) 9g
Caulis Trachelospermi (*Luo Shi Teng*) 5g
Myrrha (*Mo Yao*) 5g
Pericarpium Citri Reticulatae (*Chen Pi*) 5g
Fructus Immaturus citri Seu Ponciri (*Zhi Shi*) 5g
fresh Fructus Crataegi (*Shan Zha*) 9g

For the upper extremity use:

Ramulus Mori Albi (*Sang Zhi*) 9g

For the lower extremity use:

Radix Achyranthis Bidentatae (*Niu Xi*) 9g

All [of the above medicinals] fulfill the purpose of quickening the blood and transforming stasis, dispersing swelling and arresting pain. Once the swelling has subsided, measures are aimed at harmonizing the constructive/*ying* and knitting the bone. Therefore, the following medicinals are administered:

Radix Angelicae Sinensis (*Dang Gui*) 10g
Radix Rubrus Paeoniae Lactiflorae (*Chi Shao*) 5g
Rhizoma Ligustici Wallichii (*Chuan Xiong*) 5g

Flos Carthami Tinctorii (*Hong Hua*) 5g
Rhizoma Drynariae (*Gu Sui Bu*) 5g
Pyritum (*Zi Ran Tong*) 9g
Fructus Sambucudis (*Shuo Zhuo Zi*) 9g
Caulis Milletiae Seu Spatholobi (*Ji Xue Teng*) 9g
Pericarpium Citri Reticulatae (*Chen Pi*) 5g
Fructus Immaturus Citri Seu Ponciri (*Zhi Shi*) 5g

For the upper limbs add:

Ramulus Mori Albi (*Sang Zhi*) 10g
Lignum Pini Nodi (*Song Jie*) 9g

For the lower limbs add:

Radix Achyranthis Bidentatae (*Niu Xi*) 5g
Radix Acanthopanacis (*Wu Jia Pi*) 9g

Moving into the next stage, Pyritum and Flos Carthami Tinctorii are deleted and the following medicinals are added, as the treatment measures shift from "purging and harmonizing" to "supplementing and harmonizing":

Radix Dipsaci (*Xu Duan*) 9g
Radix Rehmanniae (*Sheng Di*) 9g

After severe bone fractures of the extremities in geriatric patients or in the latter stages of healing, atrophy of the tissues of the limbs is commonly observed, as well as adhesions, delayed recovery time and, in extreme cases, incomplete unions at the site of the fracture. These are due to a weakness of both the liver and kidney, insufficiency of the qi and blood resulting in malnutrition of the sinew and bone. Therefore, [the following medicinals] are typically employed:

Radix Codonopsis Pilosulae (*Dang Shen*) 10g
raw Radix Astragali Seu Hedysari (*Huang Qi*) 9g
Radix Angelicae Sinensis (*Dang Gui*) 9g
Radix Albus Paeoniae Lactiflorae (*Bai Shao*) 6g
Rhizoma Ligustici Wallichii (*Chuan Xiong*) 5g
Radix Dipsaci (*Xu Duan*) 9g
Semen Psoraleae Corylifoliae (*Bu Gu Zhi*) 9g
Cortex Eucommiae Ulmoidis (*Du Zhong*) 9g
Fructus Lycii Chinensis (*Gou Qi*) 5g
Frucutus Seu Semen Amomi (*Sha Ren*) 2g
Radix Saussureae Seu Vladimiriae (*Mu Xiang*) 5g

In the case of yin vacuity, add:

Radix Polygoni Multiflori (*He Shou Wu*) 9g
Carapax Amydae (*Bie Jia*) 12g

In the case yang vacuity, add:

Herba Cistanchis (*Rou Cong Rong*) 9g
Cornu Cervi Parvum (*Lu Rong*) 9g

[These medicinals] enrich and supplement the liver and kidney, benefit the qi, and nourish the blood.

For the upper extremities add:

Ramulus Mori Albi (*Sang Zhi*) 10g

For the lower extremities add:

Radix Achyranthis Bidentatae (*Niu Xi*) 9g

In areas of the trunk pressing close to the organs and viscera, following bone fractures there are typically internal injuries. The ribs are close to the lungs and heart internally and, with the dividing line of the liver channel, a fracture of the ribs will cause obstruction of the blood and result in a lack of perfusion of the lung qi and liver qi constraint. [Symptoms such as] thoraco-costal oppression and pain, respiratory inhibition and cough, expectoration and rough breathing are typically seen. [Medicinals] typically used are:

Radix Angelicae Sinensis (*Dang Gui*) 10g
Radix Rubrus Paeoniae Lactiflorae (*Chi Shao*) 10g
Rhizoma Ligustici Wallichii (*Chuan Xiong*) 6g
Semen Pruni Persicae (*Tao Ren*) 9g
Lignum Sappanis (*Su Mu*) 9g
Rhizoma Corydalis Yanhusuo (*Yan Hu Suo*) 9g
Pericarpium Viridis Citri Reticulatae (*Qing Pi*) 5g
Fructus Immaturus Citri Seu Ponciri (*Zhi Shi*) 5g
Fructus Perillae Frutescentis (*Su Zi*) 6g
Fructus Trichosanthis Kirlowii (*Gua Lou*) entire fruit, 9g
Tuber Curcumae (*Yu Jin*) 9g
raw Fructus Crataegi (*Shan Zha*) 9g

All [of the above medicinals] fulfill the purpose of transforming stasis, perfusing lung qi, and transforming phlegm.

With the presence of heat, add:

Radix Bupleuri (*Chai Hu*) 5g
Radix Salviae Miltiorrhizae (*Dan Shen*) 9g

With phlegm stagnating the blood or severe pain, add:

Radix Pseudoginseng (*San Qi*) powdered, 2g

With heart pain and emesis, add:

Yu Dan Compound (available in patent form) 1g
raw Haematitum (*Dai Zhe Shi*) 15g
Flos Inulae (*Xuan Fu Hua*) 9g

With dyspnea, add:

Semen Tinglizi (*Ting Li Zi*) 5g

During the middle stage, treatment measures of quickening the blood and knitting the bones, perfusing the lung and regulating the qi are indicated. The medicinals employed are:

Apex Radicis Angelicae Sinensis (*Gui Wei*) 9g
Radix Rubrus Paeoniaeae Lactiflorae (*Chi Shao*) 6g
Rhizoma Ligustici Wallichii (*Chuan Xiong*) 6g
Flos Carthami Tinctorii (*Hong Hua*) 5g
Herba Lycopi Lucidi (*Ze Lan*) 5g
Pyritum (*Zi Ran Tong*) 9g
Eupolyphagae Seu Ophithoplatiae (*Tu Bie Chong*) 9g
Tuber Curcumae (*Yu Jin*) 9g
Rhizoma Corydalis Yanhusuo (*Yan Hu Suo*) 9g
Pericarpium Viridis Citri Reticulatae (*Qing Pi*) 5g
Fructus Perillae Frutescentis (*Su Zi*) 5g
Fructus Trichosanthis Kirlowii (*Gua Lou*) entire fruit, 5g
Semen Pruni Persicae (*Tao Ren*) 9g
Semen Pruni Armeniacae (*Xing Ren*) 9g
Pericarpium Citri Reticulatae (*Chen Pi*) 9g

After four to five weeks the fracture will have been knitted. If there is pain upon deep respiration and severe pain when coughing, then use:

Radix Angelicae Sinensis (*Dang Gui*) 9g
Rhizoma Ligusticii Wallichi (*Chuan Xiong*) 5g
Herba Lycopi Lucidi (*Ze Lan*) 5g

Pericarpium Viridis Citri Reticulatae (*Qing Pi*) 9g
Pericarpium Citri Reticulatae (*Chen Pi*) 9g
Tuber Curcumae (*Yu Jin*) 9g
Rhizoma Corydalis Yanhusuo (*Yan Hu Suo*) 6g
Radix Dipsaci (*Xu Duan*) 9g
Rhizoma Drynariae (*Gu Sui Bu*) 9g
Fructus Citri Seu Ponciri Immaturis (*Zhi Ke*) 5g
Semen Pruni Armeniacae (*Xing Ren*) 9g
Fructus Citri Sacrodactylis (*Fu Shou*) 9g

These harmonize the constructive/*ying* and regulate the qi, perfuse the lung, transform phlegm, and promote recuperation. During the latter stage of a costal fracture, caution should be exercised in using fortifying prescriptions so as to avoid an accumulation of qi and blood creating an internal stasis and promoting [further] injury.

In the case of mid-spinal fractures, in contrast to the often seen fractures to the thoracic vertebrae, the location of these fractures proximal to the middle warmer will typically result in injuries to the abdominal area. Following bone fractures in this area, constipation is commonly observed, as well as thoracic and abdominal pain. Thus, the following medicinals are typically prescribed to purge it:

raw Radix Et Rhizoma Rhei (*Da Huang*) 10g
Cortex Magnoliae Officinalis (*Hou Po*) 9g
Pulvis Radicis Glycyrrhizae treated with Soduim Sulfate (*Yuan Ming Fen*) 10g
raw Fructus Immaturus Citri Su Ponciri (*Zhi Shi*) 9g
Apex Radicis Angelicae Sinensis (*Gui Wei*) 10g
Radix Rubrus Paeoniae Lactiflorae (*Chi Shao*) 9g
Semen Pruni Persicae(*Tao Ren*) 10g
Tuber Curcumae (*Yu Jin*) 9g
Cortex Cinnamomi (*Rou Gui*) 2g

Lignum Sappanis (*Su Mu*) 9g
Radix Saussureae Seu Vladimiriae (*Mu Xiang*) 9g
Caulis Akebiae Mutong (*Mu Tong*) 5g
Radix Achyranthis Bidentatae (*Niu Xi*) 9g

Once the constipation has been dealt with, the treatment principles become those of quickening the blood and transforming stasis, benefitting the qi and knitting the bone. The following medicinals are employed:

Apex Radicis Angelicae Sinensis (*Gui Wei*) 10g
Radix Rubrus Paeoniae Lactiflorae (*Chi Shao*) 6g
Rhizoma Ligustici Wallichii (*Chuan Xiong*) 5g
Lignum Sappanis (*Su Mu*) 9g
Herba Lycopi Lucidi (*Ze Lan*) 5g
Semen Pruni Persicae (*Tao Ren*) 9g
Pyritum (*Zi Ran Tong*) 9g
Eupolyphagae Seu Ophistoplatiae (*Tu Bie Chong*) 9g
Sanguis Draconis (*Xue Jie*) 5g
Tuber Curcumae (*Yu Jin*) 9g
Rhizoma Corydalis Yanhusuo (*Yan Hu Suo*) 9g
Radix Achyranthis Bidentatae (*Niu Xi*) 5g

Eupolyphagae Seu Ophistoplatiae, Sanguis Draconis, Tuber Curcumae, and Rhizoma Corydalis Yanhusuo should then be deleted and the following medicinals employed so as to shift from purgation to supplementation:

Rhizoma Drynariae (*Gu Sui Bu*) 9g
Radix Dipsaci (*Xu Duan*) 9g
Rhizoma Cibotii (*Gou Ji*) 9g
Apex Radicis Angelicae Sinensis (*Gui Wei*) 10g
Radix Achyranthis Bidentatae (*Niu Xi*) 5g

After five or six weeks, use the following medicinals to enrich and supplement the liver and kidney, benefit the qi, nourish the blood, and promote rapid recuperation:

Radix Codonopsis Pilosulae (*Dang Shen*) 10g
Radix Astragali Seu Hedysari (*Huang Qi*) 10g
cooked Radix Rehmanniae (*Sheng Di*) 10g
Radix Angelicae Sinensis (*Dang Gui*) 10g
Rhizoma Atractylodis Macrocephalae (*Bai Zhu*) 6g
Radix Albus Paeoniae Lactiflorae (*Bai Shao*) 6g
Rhizoma Ligustici Wallichii (*Chuan Xiong*) 5g
Fructus Lycii Chinensis (*Gou Qi Zi*) 9g
Fructus Psoraleae Corylifoliae (*Bu Gu Zhi*) 5g
Cortex Eucommiae Ulmoidis (*Du Zhong*) 10g
Ramus Loranthi Seu Visci (*Sang Ji Sheng*) 9g
Pericarpium Citri Reticulatae (*Chen Pi*) 5g
Radix Saussureae Seu Vladimiriae (*Mu Xiang*) 3g

Case Histories

The following case histories are by Shi Yang-shan, a well known specialist in the treatment of bone fractures. They were recorded by Shi Yang-shan and arranged by Qian Jin-le. They exemplify the use of medicinal substances with manual techniques in the treatment and cure of bone fractures.

Case 1: Fracture of the superior epicondyle of the humerus

Patient Qiu, an 8 year old child

Initial consultation: March 22, 1962

Main complaint: The patient fell and incurred a fragmented fracture at the lower extremity of the superior epicondyle of the humerus.

Diagnostic examination: [Examination revealed] injury to the sinew and blood vessels, congelation and accumulation of blood stasis, prolonged swelling, soreness, and pain, inability to move the [the effected arm], and such a severe injury to the joint that there was deformity.

Treatment measures: First reduce and set [the fracture], then apply a binding for the transformation of stasis.

Prescription:

Herba Seu Flos Schizonepetae Tenuifoliae (*Jing Jie Sui*) 2 *qian*
Radix Ledebouriellae Sesloidis (*Fang Feng*) 2 *qian*
burnt Fructus Gardeniae Jasminoidis (*Zhi Zi*) 2 *qian*
Radix Rehmanniae (*Sheng Di*) 4 *qian*
baked Eupolyphagae Seu Ophistolpatiae (*Tu Bie Chong*) 2 *qian*
processed Rhizoma Arisaematis (*Nan Xing*) 1 1/2 *qian*
Lignum Sappanis (*Su Mu*) 2 *qian*
Herba Lycopi Lucidi (*Ze Lan*) 3 *qian*
northern Radix Rubrus Paeoniae Lactiflorae (*Chi Shao*) 3 *qian*
Semen Vaccariae Segetalis (*Wang Bu Liu Xing*) 3 *qian*
calcined Pyritum (*Zi Ran Tong*) 4 *qian*, wrapped
baked Gummum Olibani (*Ru Xiang*) 1 *qian*
Semen Pruni Persicae (*Tao Ren*) 3 *qian*
Feces Trogopterori Seu Pteromi (*Wu Ling Zhi*) 1 piece, wrapped

Second visit: March 24. The fragmented fracture at the lower extremity of the superior epicondyle of the humerus had stabilized. [However], after being set the there was some transformation of blood stasis. [Additionally], the swelling and pain had scattered in all directions, extending to the shoulder joint and into the fingers. [The patient] was unable to move [the effected limb] and there was severe injury to the [elbow] joint. Again, [the treatment measures were] to transform stasis and dissipate swelling, knit the bone, and extinguish pain.

Prescription:

Radix Ledebouriellae Sesloidis (*Fang Feng*) 1 1/2 *qian*
baked Eupolyphagae Seu Ophistoplatiae (*Tu Bie Chong*) 2 *qian*
prepared Rhizoma Arisaematis (*Nan Xing*) 1 1/2 *qian*
Radix Angelicae Duhuo (*Du Huo*) 1 1/2 *qian*
Radix Rehmanniae (*Sheng Di*) 4 *qian*
northern Radix Rubrus Paeoniae Lactiflorae (*Chi Shao*) 3 *qian*
Herba Lycopi Lucidi (*Ze Lan*) 3 *qian*
sliced Rhizoma Curcumae (*Jiang Huang*) 1 1/2 *qian*
Semen Vaccariae Segetalis (*Wang Bu Liu Xing*) 3 *qian*
calcined Pyritum (*Zi Ran Tong*) 4 *qian*, wrapped
Rhizoma Drynariae (*Gu Sui Bu*) 3 *qian*
charred Gummum Olibani (*Ru Xiang*) 1 *qian*
Myrrha (*Mo Yao*) 1 *qian*
powdered Cortex Radicis Moutan (*Dan Pi*) 2 *qian*
Semen Pruni Persicae (*Tao Ren*) 3 *qian*

Third visit: March 27th. The fragmented fracture at the lower extremity of the superior epicondyle of the humerus had stabilized and, after being set, there was some gradual transformation of the blood stasis. The swelling and pain had also diminished, however, there was a sensation of soreness and numbness in the finger joints. [The treatment] plan was to quicken the blood, soothe the sinew, and knit the bone.

Prescription:

Radix Ledebouriellae Sesloidis (*Fang Feng*) 1 1/2 *qian*
baked Eupolyphagae Seu Ophistoplatiae (*Tu Bie Chong*) 2 *qian*

prepared Rhizoma Arisaematis (*Nan Xing*) 1 1/2 *qian*
Caulis Et Folium Lonicerae (*Jen Tong Teng*) 1 1/2 *qian*
northern Radix Rubrus Paeoniae Lactiflorae (*Chi Shao*) 3 *qian*
Radix Rehmanniae (*Sheng Di*) 4 *qian*
Herba Lycopi Lucidi (*Ze Lan*) 3 *qian*
sliced Rhizoma Curcumae (*Jiang Huang*) 1 1/2 *qian*
Semen Vaccariae Segetalis (*Wang Bu Liu Xing*) 3 *qian*
calcined Pyritum (*Zi Ran Tong*) 4 *qian*, wrapped
Rhizoma Drynariae (*Gu Sui Bu*) 3 *qian*
charred Gummum Olibani (*Ru Xiang*) 1 *qian*
Semen Pruni Persicae (*Tao Ren*) 3 *qian*

Fourth visit: April 5th: The fragmented fracture at the superior epicondyle of the right humerus was gradually knitting and the swelling and pain had diminished. The bony deformity had also subsided and the soreness and numbness in the hands and fingers was gone. [Treatment measures were for] quickening the blood, soothing the sinew, and strengthening the bone.

Prescription:

Radix Ledebouriellae Sesloidis (*Fang Feng*) 1 1/2 *qian*
baked Eupolyphagae Seu Ophistoplatiae (*Tu Bie Chong*) 2 *qian*
Radix Salviae Miltiorrhizae (*Dan Shen*) 3 *qian*
Radix Angelicae Duhuo (*Du Huo*) 1 1/2 *qian*
Radix Dipsaci (*Xu Duan*) 3 *qian*
Rhizoma Cibotii (*Gou Ji*) 4 *qian*
Herba Lycopi Lucidi (*Ze Lan*) 3 *qian*
sliced Rhizoma Curcumae (*Jiang Huang*) 1 1/2 *qian*
prepared Squama Mantidis (*Chuan Shan Jia*) 1 1/2 *qian*
calcined Pyritum (*Zi Ran Tong*) 4 *qian*, wrapped
Herba Lycopodii (*Shen Jin Cao*) 4 *qian*
Semen Pruni Persicae (*Tao Ren*) 3 *qian*
raw Radix Glycyrrhizae (*Sheng Gan Cao*) 5 *fen*

Fifth visit: April 12. The fracture had essentially knit and the soreness and pain were minimal. Function [in the arm] had improved and the prescription was changed to a dispersing formulae.

Commentary: In the treatment of this pediatric fracture of the superior epicondyle of the humerus, chief in the course of treatment is the reduction of the deformity. This is appropriately done with the topical application of stabilization [techniques]. [Proper] pattern discrimination in the internal administration of medicinal substances also enables speedy resolution of the rapid onset of stasis and swelling, and a quick healing of the bone fracture itself. In this case, aside from the general use of medicinals for transforming stasis, reducing swelling, setting the bone, and knitting the sinew in the early stage of the fracture, medicinals for clearing heat and cooling the blood, such as Cortex Radicis Moutan, Fructus Gardeniae Jasminoidis, Radix Rehmanniae, and Cauli Et Foliums Lonicerae were administered to allay any worry that the blood stasis would transform into heat. Serious fractures are typically accompanied by the expression of such global symptoms as fever, aversion to cold, torpid intake, floating and rapid pulse. This is a result of blood stasis in the channels and connecting vessels and loss of harmony between the constructive and defensive [qi]. Master Shi is expert in the use of Herba Seu Flos Schizonepetae Tenuifoliae, Radix Ledebouriellae Sesloidis, and Rhizoma Arisaematis to harmonize the constructive/*ying* and course the surface, disperse binding, and arrest pain.

In clinical observation, the inclusion of the above medicinals in blood quickening, stasis transforming prescriptions, courses and unblocks the qi and blood at both the surface and the interior. Additionally, [these medicinals] rapidly transport the blood, dispersing stasis heat and obstructive swelling, yielding a clear therapeutic effect.

[Translators note: the "manual techniques" noted in the title of Case 1 were not specified. One can assume that they consisted of the standard measures for reducing a fracture of this kind.]

Case 2: Prolonged non-union of fractures at the lower segments of the tibia and fibula.

Patient Chen You, 24 years old

Initial visit: February 5, 1958

Main complaint: [The patient suffered] fractures at the lower segment of the left tibia and fibula. It had already been in a cast for more than two months. According to the patient, X-rays revealed a non-union [fracture].

Pattern discrimination: Although the swelling appeared reduced, the tibia was sore, feeble, and lacked strength. A long period of time had passed without a union due to the weakened state of the patient.

Treatment measures: The plan was to harmonize the blood and generate the new, fortify the sinew and strengthen the bone, in the hope of reversing the situation.

Prescription:

Radix Angelica Sinensis (*Quan Dang Gui*) 3 *qian*
baked Gummum Olibani (*Ru Xiang*) 1 *qian*
Rhizoma Ligustici Wallichii (*Chuan Xiong*) 1 *qian*
Radix Achyranthis Bidentatae (*Niu Xi*) 4 *qian*
Radix Dipsaci (*Xu Duan*) 4 *qian*
Herba Lycopi Lucidi (*Ze Lan*) 1 1/2 *qian*
baked Eupolyphagae Seu Ophistoplatiae (*Tu Bie Chong*) 2 *qian*
Rhizoma Drynariae (*Gu Sui Bu*) 1 1/2 *qian*

powdered Cortex Radicis Moutan (*Dan Pi*) 1/2 *qian*
Sclerotium Poriae Cocoris (*Fu Ling*) 4 *qian*
Ramulus Mori Albi (*Sang Zhi*) 4 *qian*
calcined Pyritum (*Zi Ran Tong*) 4 *qian*

Second visit: February 8th. Following administration of the stabilizing medicinals, the skeletal structure in the region of the fracture had become somewhat more smooth. The previous treatment measures were thus deemed appropriate.

Prescription:

Radix Angelicae Sinensis (*Quan Dang Gui*) 3 *qian*
baked Eupolyphagae Seu Ophistoplatiae (*Tu Bie Chong*) 1 1/2 *qian*
Rhizoma Ligustici Wallichii (*Chuan Xiong*) 1 *qian*
burnt Rhizoma Atractylodis Macrocephalae (*Bai Zhu*) 2 *qian*
baked Gummum Olibani (*Ru Xiang*) 1 *qian*
Herba Lycopi Lucidi (*Ze Lan*) 1/2 *qian*
Radix Achyranthis Bidentatae (*Niu Xi*) 4 *qian*
Radix Dipsaci (*Xu Duan*) 4 *qian*
Rhizoma Drynariae (*Gu Sui Bu*) 1 1/2 *qian*, hairs removed
powdered Cortex Radicis Moutan (*Dan Pi*) 1/2 *qian*
Ramulus Mori Albi (*Sang Zhi*) 4 *qian*
calcined Pyritum (*Zi Ran Tong*) 4 *qian*

Third visit: February 14. Upon administration of therapy to the fracture, both components appeared to have knit. [The patient], however, experienced some turbidity during urination. The treatment plan was aimed toward banking the root and securing the source, quickening the blood, and strengthening the bone.

Prescription:

fried Radix Codonopsis Pilosulae (*Dang Shen*) 2 *qian*

Radix Achyranthis Bidentatae (*Niu Xi*) 4 *qian*
Rhizoma Ligustici Wallichi (*Chuan Xiong*) 1 *qian*
burnt Rhizoma Atractylodis Macrocephalae (*Bai Zhu*) 2 *qian*
baked Gummum Olibani (*Ru Xiang*) 1 *qian*
Herba Lycopi Lucidi (*Ze Lan*) 1 1/2 *qian*
Radix Angelicae Sinensis (*Dang Gui*) 2 *qian*
Radix Dipsaci (*Xu Duan*) 3 *qian*
Rhizoma Drynariae (*Gu Sui Bu*)1 1/2 *qian*
Rhizoma Alismatis (*Ze Xie*) 3 *qian*
Ramulus Mori Albi (*Sang Zhi*) 4 *qian*
calcined Pyritum (*Zi Ran Tong*) 3 *qian*

Fourth visit: February 21. Two months after the fracture and following [the above] course of therapy, the fracture appeared to have smoothed out and bone knitting was evident. The urination had cleared. Here there was some divergence from the original plan.

Prescription:

Radix Angelicae Sinensis (*Dang Gui*) 3 *qian*
fried Rhizoma Atractylodis Macrocephalae (*Bai Zhu*) 3 *qian*
Radix Dioscoreae Oppositae (*Shan Yao*) 3 *qian*
burnt Rhizoma Atractylodis (*Cang Zhu*) 2 *qian*
Radix Dipsaci (*Xu Duan*) 4 *qian*
fried Rhizoma Alismatis (*Ze Xie*) 4 *qian*
Radix Achyranthis Bidentatae (*Niu Xi*) 4 *qian*
Rhizoma Drynariae (*Gu Sui Bu*) 1 1/2 *qian*, hairs removed
Rhizoma Ligustici Wallichi (*Chuan Xiong*) 1 *qian*
powdered Cortex Radicis Moutan (*Dan Pi*) 1/2 *qian*
Sclerotium Poriae Cocoris (*Fu Ling*) 4 *qian*
Ramulus Mori Albi (*Sang Zhi*) 4 *qian*
calcined Pyritum (*Zi Ran Tong*) 4 *qian*

Fifth visit: February 28. With treatment, the fracture of the lower segments of the tibia and fibula had essentially knitted. However, the patient remained in a weakened condition. Treatment was aimed at regulating and supplementing. Two *liang* of both ***Zi Shen Wan*** and ***Jian Bu Hu Qian Wan*** divided over seven days were administered orally with boiled water.

Commentary: In this fracture of the lower segments of the tibia and fibula, since the blood supply was relatively poor, healing was also relatively slow. An insufficiency of qi and blood within the liver and kidney will often result in impaired bone knitting as well. Xiao-shan has had considerable treatment experience with patients suffering from prolonged non-union fractures, and over the years has been quite successful in treating [this condition]. He has recognized that in this pattern, the essential cause is an essence vacuity producing an inability to irrigate [the bones], a blood vacuity causing an inability to moisten and nourish, and qi vacuity causing an inability to warm. Treatment is, therefore, most appropriately discussed from the perspective of vacuity and depletion. In prescription composition in general, augmentation of the liver and kidney, nourishment of the qi and blood, and filling in the essence marrow cannot be deviated from. This enables nourishment of the [fractured] ends and facilitates a complete recovery. Occasionally, Colla Cornu Cervi (*Lu Jiao Jiao*) or Os Tigridis (*Hu Gu*) is added to the above prescription. (In modern times, supplies of Os Tigridis are insufficient, and monkey bones are commonly used in its place). Colla Cornu Cervi has an affinity for the flesh and blood. It is used because of it's form to fortify form. By this it is meant that [Cornu Cervi and bone] have similar natures. [Colla Cornu Cervi] additionally assists in the regulatory aspect of therapy by quickening the blood and unblocking the collaterals, and is especially helpful in blood transportation to the fracture sight. Considerable attention should be paid to external treatment as well, with external application of medicinals such as *Shang Gao*[8] and *Jie Gu Dan* (an empirical prescription of Master Shi) which adopts both internal emolliating and external hardening components in bringing stabilization.

Case 3: Fractured rib

Patient Gu, 30 years old.

Initial visit: February 28, 1959

Main complaint: [The patient] experienced intense soreness and pain following an injury five days previously. To protect his respiration, he would shift onto his side. *Qi Li San* was administered internally and *Shang Gao* was administered topically. However, the pain increased daily. There was, concomitantly, a choking cough with rough respiration and inhibited bowel movements.

---

8 *Zhong Yi Shang Ke Xue (The Study of Traditional Chinese Traumatology)*, a standard textbook on traumatology published by the Shanghai Science & Technology Press, contains a prescription which, while most probably not precisely the *Shang Gao* mentioned above, is certainly analogous.

Shang You Gao: Sanguis Draconis (*Xue Jie*) 60g, Flos Carthami Tinctorii (*Hong Hua*) 6g, Gummum Olibani (*Ru Xiang*) 6g, Myrrha (*Mo Yao*) 6g, Acacia Catechu (*Er Cha*) 6g, Succinum (*Hu Po*) 3g, Borneolum (*Bing Pian*) 3g, added last, Sesame oil 1500g, Honey, an appropriate amount

This quickens the blood and arrests pain. It is most often used by applying it to the affected area when using manual techniques, as it simultaneously achieves a moistening effect. Preparation: With the exception of the Borneolum, sesame oil, and honey, grind the ingredients into a fine powder, adding the Borneolum last. Fry these in the sesame oil, finally adding in the honey to form a paste.

Examination: Palpation of the 7th, 8th, and 9th ribs revealed a sound of bones rubbing [against one another]. The tongue had a slimy, thin coat and the pulse was wiry and a little tense.

Treatment measures: The initial plan was to transform stasis and normalize the qi, harmonize the collaterals and arrest pain.

Prescription:

Apex Radicis Angelicae Sinensis (*Gui Wei*) 4 *qian*
baked Eupolyphagae Seu Ophistoplatiae (*Tu Bie Chong*) 3 *qian*
Radix Salviae Miltiorrhizae (*Dan Shen*) 3 *qian*
baked Gummum Olibani (*Ru Xiang*) 1/2 *qian*
baked Myrrha (*Mo Yao*) 1/2 *qian*
prepared Rhizoma Cyperi Rotundi (*Xiang Fu*) 3 *qian*
Exocarpium Citri Rubri (*Ju Hong*) 1 *qian*
Fasciculus Vascularis Luffae (*Si Gua Luo*) 1 *qian*
Semen Pruni Armeniacae (*Xing Ren*) 4 *qian*
Semen Pruni Persicae (*Tao Ren*) 4 *qian*
Flos Inulae (*Xuan Fu Hua*) 3 *qian*, wrapped
Semen Sinapis Albae (*Bai Jie Zi*) 1/2 *qian*
sliced Lignum Aquilariae Agallochae (*Chen Xiang*) 8 *fen*
powdered Radix Pseudoinseng (*San Qi*) swallowed [separately]
Li Dong Wan, 1 piece, swallowed [seperately]

A cardboard liner [over the affected area] and bound to the body with numerous wraps was used for the topical application of medicinals for transforming stasis and knitting the bone.

Second visit: March 3rd. Following [topical] application and [internal] administration of the medicinals for the fractures of the right ribs, there was some transformation of stasis and the respiration had become somewhat more smooth. The injured area protruded slightly, and the sound of bones grating remained. [The patient suffered from] a hacking cough causing a drawing pain, and was not sleeping restfully at night. Again the original prescription was used with the addition of a few [medicinals] in the class of settling the spirit.

Prescription:

Apex Radicis Angelicae Sinensis (*Dang Gui*) 4 *qian*
baked Eupolyphagae Seu ophistoplatiae (*Tu Bie Chong*) 3 *qian*
Radix Salviae Miltiorrhizae (*Dan Shen*) 3 *qian*
baked Gummum Olibani (*Ru Xiang*) 1/2 *qian*
baked Myrrha (*Mo Yao*) 1/2 *qian*
Pericarpium Citri Rubri (*Ju Hong*) 1 *qian*
Fasciculus Vascularis Luffae (*Si Gua Luo*) 1 *qian*
Flos Inulae (*Xuan Fu Hua*) 3 *qian*, wrapped
Rhizoma Corydalis Yanhusuo (*Yan Hu Suo*) 1/2 *qian*
sliced Lignum Aquilariae Agallochae (*Chen Xiang*) 8 *fen*
Sanguis Draconis (*Xue Jie*) 1 *qian*
baked Radix Polygalae Tenuifoliae (*Yuan Zhi*) 1/2 *qian*
Sclerotium Pararadicis Poriae Cocoris (*Fu Shen*) 4 *qian*

Third visit: March 6th. The grating sound had diminished at the sight of the right rib fracture. The soreness and pain which accompanied respiration and the hacking cough had lessened as well, however, the patient continued to sleep poorly. Treatment was again aimed at transforming stasis and rectifying the qi, harmonizing the collaterals and settling the spirit.

Prescription:

Apex Radicis Angelicae Sinensis (*Gui Wei*) 4 *qian*
baked Eupolyphagae Seu Ophistoplatiae (*Tu Bie Chong*) 3 *qian*
Radix Salviae Miltiorrhizae (*Dan Shen*) 3 *qian*
baked Gummum Olibani (*Ru Xiang*) 1/2 *qian*
Semen Pruni Persicae (*Tao Ren*) 4 *qian*
Semen Pruni Armeniacae (*Xing Ren*) 4 *qian*

Flos Inulae (*Xuan Fu Hua*) 3 *qian*, wrapped
Herba Lycopodii (*Shen Jin Cao*) 2 *qian*
Rhizoma Corydalis Yanhusuo (*Yan Hu Suo*) 2 *qian*
sliced Lignum Aquilariae Agallochae (*Chen Xiang*) 8 *fen*
Rhizoma Coptidis Chinensis (*Huang Lian*) 5 *fen*
Semen Zizyphi Spinosae (*Suan Zao Ren*) 3 *qian*
Fructus Citri Seu Ponciri (*Zhi Ke*) 1/2 *qian*, baked
Fasciculus Vascularis Luffae (*Si Gua Luo*) 3 *qian*

Fourth visit: March 11th. With treatment, the qi stasis at the site of the fracture had gradually normalized and transformed and there was some initial congelation and knitting of the bone. The cough had stabilized and the pain had diminished as well. Sleep had improved only slightly and he was still uncomfortable when shifting onto his side. [Treatment measures were] again to quicken the blood and rectify the qi, knit the bone and settle the spirit.

Prescription:

Radix Angelicae Sinensis (*Quan Dang Gui*) 3 *qian*
Cortex Eucommiae Ulmoidis (*Du Zhong*) 4 *qian*, fried in salt water
Radix Dipsaci (*Xu Duan*) 4 *qian*
baked Eupolyphagae Seu Ophistoplatiae (*Tu Bie Chong*) 3 *qian*
Rhizoma Corydalis Yanhusuo (*Yan Hu Suo*) 2 *qian*
Sanguis Draconis (*Xue Jie*) 1 *qian*
sliced Lignum Aquilariae Agallochae (*Chen Xiang*) 8 *fen*
Pericarpium Viridis Citri Reticulatac (*Qing Pi*) 1 *qian*
Pericarpium Citri Reticulatae (*Chen Pi*) 1 *qian*
baked Radix Polygalae Tenuifoliae (*Yuan Zhi*) 1/2 *qian*
Cortex Albizziae (*He Huan Pi*) 3 *qian*

Fifth visit: After being treated four times for the fractures of the right ribs, the skeletal structure had basically knit. The patient would cough when shifting onto his side and although the grating sound had ceased, a drawing pain persisted. His sleep remained unsettled and he took no pleasure in eating. The plan was to harmonize the blood and regulate the qi, settle the spirit and please the stomach.

Prescription:

Radix Angelicae Sinensis (*Quan Dang Gui*) 2 *qian*
Radix Rubrus Paeoniae Lactiflorae (*Chi Shao*) 3 *qian*
Radix Albus Paeoniae Lactiflorae (*Bai Shao*) 3 *qian*
Radix Salviac Miltiorrhizae (*Dan Shen*) 3 *qian*
Radix Dipsaci (*Xu Duan*) 3 *qian*
Rhizoma Corydalis Yanhusuo (*Yan Hu Suo*) 2 *qian*
Rhizoma Cyperi Rotundi (*Xiang Fu*) 2 *qian*
Rhizoma Pinelliae Ternatae (*Ban Xia*) 1/2 *qian*
sliced Fructus Citri Sacrodactylis (*Fu Shou*) 2 *qian*
Fructus Germinatus Hordei Vulgaris (*Mai Ya*) 4 *qian*
Fructus Germinatus Oryzae Sativae (*Gu Ya*) 4 *qian*
husked Sorghum (*Shu Mi*), 4 *qian*, wrapped
Medulla Junci Effusae (*Deng Cao*) 3 bundles
Sclerotim Pararadicis Poriae Cocoris (*Fu Shen*) 4 *qian*

Sixth visit: The knitting of the fractured rib had not consolidated and shifting onto side with back bent still produced drawing pain, palpitations, and poor sleep. Treatment was aimed at harmonizing the blood and generating the new, rectifying the qi and settling the spirit.

Prescription:

Radix Angelicae Sinensis (*Quan Dang Gui*) 4 *qian*
Radix Rubrus Paeoniae Lactiflorae (*Chi Shao*) 3 *qian*
Radix Albus Paeoniae Lactiflorae (*Bai Shao*) 3 *qian*
Radix Salviae Miltiorrhizae (*Dan Shen*) 3 *qian*

fried Cortex Eucommiae Ulmoidis (*Du Zhong*) 4 *qian*
Ramus Loranthi Seu Visci (*Sang Ji Sheng*) 4 *qian*
Rhizoma Corydalis Yanhusuo (*Yan Hu Suo*) 2 *qian*
Radix Rehmanniae (*Sheng Di*) 2 *qian*
Semen Zizyphi Spinosae (*Zao Ren*) 2 *qian*
Fructus Levis Tritici (*Fu Xiao Mai*) 4 *qian*
Radix Praeparatus Glycyrrhizae (*Zhi Gan Cao*) 1 *qian*
Fructus Ziziphi Jujubae (*Da Zao*) 5 pieces
Flos Rosae Rugosae (*Mei Gui Hua*) 8 *fen*
Medulla Junci Effusae (*Deng Cao*) 3 bundles

Seventh visit: The knitting of the bone was gradually reinforced and the soreness and pain ceased. The patient could shift onto his side with relative comfort and his sleep also improved. There was some slight mental dizziness when arising from a sitting position. Following such an injury, the body has been weakened, so measures for regulating the qi and blood and banking up the source were employed.

Prescription:

Radix Angelicae Sinensis (*Quan Dang Gui*) 2 *qian*
Rhizoma Atractylodis Macrocephalae (*Bai Zhu*) 3 *qian*
Radix Albus Paeoniae Lactiflorae (*Bai Shao*) 3 *qian*
fried Radix Codonopsis Pilosulae (*Dang Shen*) 3 *qian*
fried Cortex Eucommiae Ulmoidis (*Du Zhong*) 4 *qian*
Radix Dipsaci (*Xu Duan*) 3 *qian*
Radix Rehmanniae (*Sheng Di*) 4 *qian*
Sclerotium Poriae Cocoris (*Fu Ling*) 4 *qian*
Radix Praeparatus Glycyrrhizae (*Zhi Gan Cao*) 8 *fen*
Semen Zizyphi Spinosae (*Zao Ren*) 3 *qian*
Fructus Levis Tritici (*Fu Xiao Mai*) 4 *qian*
Fructus Seu Semen Amomi (*Sha Ren*) 8 *fen*, added at the end
Er Zhi Wan, 4 *qian*, wrapped [*i.e.*, Fructus Ligustri Lucidi (*Nu Zhen Zi*) and Herba Ecliptae Prostratae (*Han Lian Cao*)]

Commentary: This [is a] case of rib fracture due to a violent external force resulting in an injury to the qi and blood. Aside from the expression of blood stasis symptoms such as soreness and pain and rough respiration, there is a loss of regulatory function within the organs and bowels as well. Cough and expectoration, torpid intake, difficult bowel [movements], palpitations, and restless sleep therefore, appear concomitantly. While the transformation of stasis and rectification of qi, bone knitting, and analgesia are of primary importance, simultaneous treatment aimed at regulating the function of the organs and bowels is nonetheless indicated, and should not be ignored. During the Qing Dynasty, Shen Ji-nao stated:

> It must be understood that injury to the exterior will produce an internal illness, and, in treating this, measures must include both the channels and connecting vessels and the organs and bowels.

Appendix

Ingredients for Bone Fracture Formulas

Wan Liu Dan*, aka *Bao An Wan Liu Dan

Rhizoma Atractylodis Macrocephalae (*Bai Zhu*)
Buthus Martensi (*Quan Xie*)
Herba Dendrobii (*Shi Hu*)
Rhizoma Gastrodia Elatae (*Tian Ma*)
Radix Angelicae Sinensis (*Dang Gui*)
Radix Glycyrrhizae (*Gan Cao*)
RHizoma Ligustici Wallichi (*Chuan Xiong*)
Radix Et Rhizoma Notoptergyii (*Qiang Huo*)
Herba Seu Flos Schizonepetae Tenuifoliae (*Jing Jie Sui*)
Radix Ledebouriellae Sesloidis (*Fang Feng*)
Herba Ephedrae (*Ma Huang*)
Herba Cum Radice Asari Sieboldi (*Xi Xin*)
Radix Aconiti (*Wu Tou*)
Radix Aconiti Cao Wu (*Cao Wu*)
Radix Polygoni Multiflori (*He Shou Wu*)

Li Dong Wan

Radix Pseudoginseng (*San Qi*)
Radix Et Rhizoma Rhei (*Da Huang*)
Resina Ferulae (*A Wei*)
Semen Acacia Catechu (*Bing Lang*)
Concretio Siliceae Bambusae (*Tian Zhu Huang*)
Sanguis Draconis (*Xue Jie*)
Gummum Olibani (*Ru Xiang*)
Myrrha (*Mo Yao*)
Realgar (*Xiong Dan*)
Borneolum (*Bing Pian*)

Secretio Moschi Moschiferi (*She Xiang*)
Calculus Bovis (*Niu Huang*)

ACCIDENTS WILL HAPPEN

Pediatric Diarrhea

Introduction

Diarrhea is one of the most common complaints presented to the pediatric practitioner. Here again, as in the chapter on hypertension, there is family of patterns common to all approaches to diagnosis and treatment. In this case, it is vacuity of spleen qi which is at the center of most cases of pediatric diarrhea. Skillful adaptation to the transformations and permutations of this central pattern can determine whether the therapy is a success or failure. In the following essays, Xu Di-san provides a general overview of his experience in treating acute and chronic infantile diarrhea, Xu Xiao-zhou presents ***Shen Ling Bai Zhu San*** and ***Shan Zha Wan*** as the primary formulas for treating pediatric diarrhea, and Meng Zhong-fa emphasizes the importance of food stagnation and proper diet in the etiology and treatment of this disorder. The case history by Wang Yu-run reflects the skillful integration of measures for treating food damage diarrhea with measures for astringing and supplementing the intestines. Gu Wen-hua's case history provides us with an example of the use of ***Chi Shi Zhi Yu Yu Liang Wan*** in the treatment of pediatric diarrhea. Xu Di-san elucidates his previous comments with a case history of his own and some comments on the parameters for the use of Pericarpium Papaveris Somniferi (*Ying Su Ke*). Finally, I have included some of my own thoughts on the issue of administering Chinese medicinals to children.

Theoretical Discussions

Xu Di-san [I]

Infantile diarrhea can be divided into two stages: acute and chronic. Acute phase diarrhea has an acute onset, the course of the illness is of short duration, and is most often violent. It typically manifests as [patterns of] cold diarrhea, heat diarrhea, and food damage diarrhea which are all due to a repletion pathogen. Since these pertain to a repletion pattern, treatment is aimed at ridding the pathogen. The condition of chronic diarrhea has a gradual onsct and the course of illness is more protracted. This is typically seen in spleen vacuity diarrhea. Being due to a vacuity of the correct qi and pertaining to a vacuity pattern in general, treatment is aimed at supporting the correct.

I. Acute diarrhea:

(1) In ridding dampness, the necessity of supplementing the spleen cannot be ignored. The primary measure in the treatment of acute diarrhea is that of ridding dampness. For instance, in cold diarrhea, measures for ridding cold and drying dampness are utilized; in heat diarrhea measures for clearing heat and disinhibiting dampness are utilized; in food damage diarrhea measures for dispersing food and transforming dampness are utilized. In all these cases, treatment proceeds with [the transformation of] dampness. External dampness precipitates a failure of the normal transportive function of the spleen, resulting in diarrhea. Thererfore, if ingredients are aimed solely at ridding dampness, then the dampness may be resolved but the transportative capacity will not be restored and the diarrhea will be difficult to cure. Sclerotium Poriae Cocoris (*Fu Ling*) and Rhizoma Atractylodis Macrocephalae (*Bai Zhu*) are, therefore, indicated to supplement the spleen and transform dampness. This will thus

hasten the recovery of the spleen's transformative function and is an important measure in the treatment of acute diarrhea.

(2) In cases of violent diarrhea measures for arresting and astringing may be used. Violent diarrhea is due to a repletion pathogen, therefore arresting and astringing measures are not customarily used during the early stages of treatment for fear that the pathogen will become lodged, prolonging the illness. Nevertheless, where there is a copious volume of violent diarrhea and there are more than ten bowel movements throughout the day and night, it is essential to minimize any damage to the yin and yang. If the correct qi is left unprotected, there will be a vacuity of the both yin and yang with undesirable ramifications. If the use of medicinals such as Pericarpium Papaveris Somniferi (*Ying Su Ke*) are considered to hinder the [expulsion of] the pathogen, then Fructus Terminaliae Chebulae (*He Zi*) and Pericarpium Punicae Graniti (*Shi Liu Pi*) can be employed. Research in modern chemistry has demonstrated the antibiotic capacities [of these medicinals]. They support the correct while ridding the pathogen and so they are ideal arresting and astringing medicinals for the treatment of acute diarrhea.

(3) The use of greasy, supplementing medicinals is not indicated if there is damage to the yin. Violent diarrhea may easily damage yin, manifesting in symptoms of water loss such as in dry mouth, dry, cracked skin, scanty urination, diminished lacrimation, and a peeled tongue. Medicinals such as Fructus Pruni Mume (*Wu Mei*) and Herba Dendrobii (*Shi Hu*) are indicated to generate fluids. The use of Radix Coquitus Rehmanniae (*Shu Di*) to nourish yin is inappropriate as it produces water dampness and a failure of transportation This only increases the burden on the spleen and stomach, which in turn aggravates the [overall] condition.

II. Chronic Diarrhea:

(1) In the case of damp papules and diarrhea it is important to employ measures for ridding dampness. In infants with longstanding damp diarrhea, rash is commonly encountered. This is characterized by diarrhea occurring simultaneously with damp papules. The illness may become drawn out, have a tendency to relapse, and be difficult to cure. This type of patient falls within the category of spleen vacuity with simultaneous dampness and heat. While the utilization of Radix Panacis Ginseng (*Ren Shen*) Sclerotium Poriae Cocoris, Rhizoma Atractylodis Macrocephalae, and Radix Glycyrrhizae (*Gan Cao*) benefits the qi and supplements the spleen, these medicinals are unable to rid dampness and heat, and more often than not fail to help the matter. The use of medicinals in the class of Spica Prunellae Vulgaris (*Xia Gu Cao*) and Cortex Radicis Dictamni (*Bai Xian Pi*) are indicated to clear and disinhibit the dampness and heat. With the dampness gone, the diarrhea is then arrested.

(2) Caution is to be exercised in the use of bitter cold medicinals for spleen vacuity diarrhea. In the case of longstanding diarrhea due to spleen vacuity, there are often symptoms of a heat pattern such as a yellow tongue coat, red tongue body, red throat, and diarrhea that seems to pour out. The use of medicinals such as Radix Scutellariae Baicalensis (*Huang Qin*) and Rhizoma Coptidis Chinensis (*Huang Lian*) to clear heat is necessary. However, bitter and cold medicinals may easily damage the spleen yang. Therefore, when their use is required, they should not be administered over an extended period of time. When there is spleen vacuity and a longstanding lodging of dampness and heat, the use of medicinals such as Flos Dolichoris[1], which

1 Semen Dolichos has the same function.

supplements the spleen while clearing and disinhibiting dampness and heat, may be appropriate.

(3) If there is a concomitant exterior [condition], then it must be treated first. During the course of chronic diarrhea, when the correct qi becomes vacuous as a result of the longstanding vacuity, there is a tendency toward recurrent external afflictions. With exterior symptoms such as fever, cough and expectoration, snivel, and a red throat, Herba Mentha (*Bo He*), Semen Praeparatus Sojae (*Dan Dou Chi*), or Folium Perillae Frutescentis (*Su Ye*) and Radix Et Rhizoma Notopterygii (*Qiang Huo*) may be employed first to course and disperse the exterior pathogen. Once the exterior has been relieved, the interior pattern will become harmonized on its own. If this does not occur and the diarrhea is not arrested, then utilization of measures for boosting the qi and strengthening the spleen can be continued, which will subsequently achieve a positive result.

Xu Xiao-zhou [I]

Pediatric diarrhea in children up to 3 years old is most commonly seen as an internal [disorder] occurring primarily in the summer and autumn. In treatment, initial attention should be paid to the regulation of the middle and the cessation of the diarrhea. If there is digestate accumulation, then [measures for] dispersing and leading [are used]. If there is dampness and heat, then [measures for] clearing and disinhibiting are used. If the diarrhea is longstanding, then [measures for] raising [the qi are used]. If there is efflux diarrhea, then [measures for] securing and containing are used. [The following are some] commonly used prescriptions for diarrhea:

(1) Prescription for pediatric diarrhea:

Radix Ledebouriellae Sesloidis (*Fang Feng*) 5g
Fructus Pruni Mume (*Wu Mei*) 5g
Radix Glycyrrhiazae (*Gan Cao*) 5g
Radix Platycodi Grandiflori (*Jie Gen*) 3g
Radix Peurariae Lobatae (*Ge Gen*) 10g
raw Fructus Crataegi (*Shan Zha*) 10g
Fructus Germinatus Hordei Vulgaris (*Mai Ya*) 10g
Fructus Germinatus Oryzae Sativae (*Gu Ya*) 10g
Dolichos husks (*Bian Dou Yi*) 10g
Radix Scutellariae Baicalensis (*Huang Qin*) 10g
Rhizoma Coptidis Chinensis (*Huang Lian*) 10g
aged Pericarpium Punicae Granati (*Shi Liu Pi*) 10g

This is indicated for diarrhea of relatively short duration, stools which are thin or foul smelling, and a thin, white or slimy tongue coat. It is indicated for use regardless of whether the diarrhea is due to an external contraction of one or more of the six environmental excesses, or to digestate damage. This prescription functions to rid wind, clear heat, supplement the spleen, and disinhibit dampness. It may nonetheless be modified according to the presenting pattern. For an exuberance of dampness and a slimy tongue coat Cortex Magnoliae Officinalis (*Hou Po*) and Herba Portulacae Oleraceae (*Ma Chi Xian*) are added. For shortened urination Sclerotium Rubrum Poriae Cocoris (*Chi Fu Ling*) and Semen Plantaginis (*Che Qian Zi*) are added. For vacuity of yang with a pale tongue, Sclerotium Poriae Cocoris (*Fu Ling*) and Rhizoma Coptidis Chinensis (*Huang Lian*) are deleted and fried Rhizoma Zingeberis (*Jiang*) and sliced Radix Praeparatus Aconiti Carmichaeli (*Fu Zi*) are added.

(2) *Shen Ling Bai Zhu San:*

Radix Codonopsis Pilosulae (*Dang Shen*) 10g

Rhizoma Atractylodis Macrocephalae (*Bai Zhu*) 10g
Sclerotium Poriae Cocoris (*Fu Ling*) 10g
Radix Glycyrrhizae (*Gan Cao*) 10g
stir-fried Rhizoma Zingeberis (*Chao Jiang*) 2g
Radix Puerariae Lobatae (*Ge Gen*) 10g
Radix Saussureae Seu Vladimiriae (*Mu Xiang*) 10g
Herba Agastachis Seu Pogostemi (*Huo Xiang*) 10g
Semen Dolichori Lablabis (*Bai Bian Dou*) 10g

This prescription is indicated for intermittent diarrhea and longstanding, intractable diarrhea. The stools are thin and undigested, the tongue moss is thin and the tongue body is pale, while the pulse is deep and lacks strength. The four sovereigns[2] in this prescription primarily supplement the qi and strengthen the spleen. With the addition of medicinals in the class of harmonizing the stomach and transforming dampness, the branch and the root are addressed simultaneously.

(3) *Tan Shan Zha Wan*

Pills of Fried Rhizoma Zingeberis, one pill each administered every 2 hours, 6 times a day. (Note: the two pills each weigh 0.3 grams). This prescription is indicated for diarrhea characterized by thin, clear stool or undigested food in the stool, with a thin, white or slimy tongue coat. The use of Fructus Crataegi (*Shan Zha*) disperses accumulated stasis; while the nature of fried Rhizoma Zingeberis is warm, protecting, and not moving. It warms the middle and arrests diarrhea. Frying the two medicinals until they are charred enhances their capacity to arrest diarrhea,

---

2 The four sovereigns are Radix Codonopsis Pilosulae, Rhizoma Atractylodes Macrocephalae, Sclerotium Poriae Cocoris, and Radix Glycyrrhizae.

and rendering them into pill form makes for convenient administration.

(4) Measures for topical application:

Pericarpium Papaveri Somniferi (*Ying Su Ke*) may be decocted down to a sap [or paste]. A gauze pad is soaked in this preparation and applied to the umbilical area, with numerous applications over the course of a day. This method is indicated for longstanding incessant diarrhea, excessive efflux diarrhea, or a failure of the stomach to assimilate. The nature of Pericarpium Papaverus is astringent and restraining and it's use topically on the umbilicus is often effective. In the case of nursing infants, when administering medication nursing should be temporarily discontinued. A decoction of millet stir fried in butter, [this is basically porridge] may be given in it's place, as this avoids prolonging the diarrhea and making it difficult to cure.

Meng Zhong-fa [I]

In discriminating patterns in pediatric diarrhea, the combination of inappropriate food and drink and a contraction of illness is commonly seen. This is usually classified as miscellaneous types of food stasis and dampness. Thus, supplementing the spleen and drying dampness are the main therapeutic measures. Longstanding diarrhea is more often than not an expression of spleen vacuity with such symptoms as a yellow face, abdominal distension, emaciation, torpid intake, fatigue, a pale tongue with a white coat, and a soggy pulse lacking strength. An accumulation of a damp pathogen in the stomach and intestines may give rise to borborygmus, thin stools, and excessive diarrhea. [Medicinals for] supplementing splenic transportation and drying dampness enhance the function of the spleen. Once the free flow of the qi dynamic has been established, the dampness and turbidity will be resolved and the stool will firm up prior to complete recovery.

Occurrences of pediatric diarrhea due to an irregular diet result mainly from a cessation of breast feeding and feeding [the infant] too much cooked rice. The child is unable to completely digest these starchy foods in the stomach and intestines. They then ferment and become sour. The stools are most often thin, sticky, yellow colored, and watery. This is accompanied by a frothy flatulence, frequent diarrhea, a reddening of the skin around the anus, borborygmus, abdominal distension, and vomiting and nausea. The tongue will be mostly white and slimy or yellow and slimy and, in general, there is no fever or a low fever. Treatment is aimed at regulating the intake of grains and substituting with foods such as soybean milk, steamed chicken, eggs, and fish. Concurrent treatment with prescriptions to digest the food and rectify the qi, dry dampness and substantiate the intestines is indicated. [Medicinals used might], for instance, include Fructus Germinatus Hordei Vulgaris, Fructus Germinatus Oryzae Sativae, raw Fructus Crateagi, Massa Medica Fermentata (*Shen Qu*), Pericarpium Citri Reticulatae (*Chen Pi*), Radix Saussureae Seu Vladimiriae, Rhizoma Coptidis Chinensis, Rhizoma Atractylodis Macrocephalae, Cortex Magnoliae Officinalis, Semen Plantaginis (*Che Qian Zi*), and Flos Dolichoris (*Bian Hua*).

Diarrhea due to contraction of an external damp heat pathogen most often pertains to viral or bacterial infection. Aside from the thin, sticky stool, a pasty, fluid stool is typically seen as well. Moreover, there will be blood and pus, and microscopic examination reveals leukocytes, erythrocytes or pyocytes, and positive bacterial cultures. There is fever, the tongue is red with a slimy, white or a slimy, yellow moss, the digital vein will be a stagnant purple color, and the pulse will be rapid. Treatment is indicated to clear heat and cleanse the bowels, supplement the spleen and rid dampness. Prescriptions such as ***Ge Gen Ling Lian Tang*** or ***Huo Xiang Zheng Qi San*** are good therapies. If there is fever, a large volume of thin stools, and the presence of leukocytes and erythrocytes is not detected, then this is likely a viral infection.

If the stools are pasty, containing pus and blood with fever and abdominal pain, then this is likely a bacterial infection. This type of infectious diarrhea is appropriate to treat with ***Hong Ling Dan, Yu Shu Dan,*** or ***Xing Jun San***, 0.1-0.2 grams taken orally 2—3 times daily. In order to achieve a definitive therapeutic effect, the diet should be regulated as well. In the case of autumnal diarrhea of a bacterial nature, ***Shu Shi Zheng Qi Wan*** may be used — 0.5-1.5 grams taken twice daily. It is generally not taken for more than a week and is quite effective. If there is dehydration, simultaneous fluid supplementation may be administered either orally or intravenously.

Protracted diarrhea is most often due to a lack of healthy bacteria in the intestinal tract resulting from extended use of antibiotics. [in which case] the immediate cessation of the use of these antibiotics is indicated. If there are symptoms of thin and foul smelling stools, diminished appetite, and emaciation ***Shen Ling Bai Zhu San*** is a key prescription. If there is a slimy, yellow tongue coat indicative of severe dampness and heat, 15-30g each of Herba Plantaginis (*Che Qian Cao*) and Herba Euphorbiae Humifusae (*Di Jin Cao*) are key ingredients. If cold and dampness is severe, then Cortex Magnoliae Officinalis, Rhizoma Zingeberis fried to a char, and Radix Praeparatus Aconiti Carmichaeli are indicated. For longstanding, incessant diarrhea, Pericarpium Citri Reticulatae, Radix Glycyrrhizae, Pericarpium Punicae Granati, and Fructus Pruni Mume may be employed to control intestinal peristalsis and to achieve the intent of astringing and arresting diarrhea. Pericarpium Citri Reticulatae and Pericarpium Punicae Granati will have dosages of 10-15g of while the dosage of Radix Glycyrrhizae should not exceed 3g, since too much will easily cause qi distension.

In the case of a child who eats and then has diarrhea, or whatever has been eaten passes in the stool with accompanying symptoms of diminished appetite and abdominal distension,

20-30g each raw Fructus Crataegi and fried Rhizoma Atractylodis Macrocephalae may be administered daily. This is cooked into a thick decoction with an appropriate amount of glucose added. Administered repeatedly by mouth, it will usually achieve the intent of arresting diarrhea and dispersing distension. On the other hand, starvation diarrhea is also a commonly encountered phenomena after the child suffers from diarrhea. The parents consequently impose excessively severe dietary restrictions. This induces a hunger condition in the child which produces intestinal peristalsis. If the child does not eat, the diarrhea will become chronic and difficult to cure.

Cases

Wang Yu-run [IV]

Infantile diarrhea

A 50 day old male.

Initial consultation: July 31, 1976. The patient was born following a normal period of gestation and a normal labor, and was bottle fed. When he was three days old he developed hemolysis which was treated effectively. Two weeks later he developed diarrhea and a local hospital used antibiotic and rehydration therapies. However, the patient continued to have 5-6 pasty bowel movements per day. In the past three days his stools had become watery, his spirits were down, and he liked to sleep [too much]. He suffered from torpid intake, nausea and vomiting, agglutinations in the eyes after sleep, and chilling of the four extremities. His fontanelle was depressed, his eyes were sunken, and he had scanty tears and nasal discharge. He had a sallow facial complexion, urgent respiration, and the upper thoracic region was obviously sunken. He had a red tongue body with little coat and a fine, rapid pulse. The pattern pertained to spleen vacuity diarrhea with a chronic loss of fluids. The treatment plan was to strengthen the spleen, augment the qi, and generate fluids.

fried Rhizoma Atractylodis Macrocephalae (*Bai Zhu*) 9g
Radix Rubrus Panacis Ginseng (*Ren Shen*) 3g
Fructus Zizyphi Jujubae (*Zao*) 15g
Fructus Pruni Mume (*Wu Mei*) 3g

This was decocted in water and small amounts were administered many times throughout the day.

In addition a 500 ml. decocted solution of fresh apple with sugar and salt was administered frequently, and a slice of raw Fructus Crataegi was administered 5 times daily. He was given skimmed milk instead of [whole] cow's milk for 4 days.

Second visit: August 2. The urgent respiration improved immediately following administration of the decoction. There was cough and expectoration with phlegm in the throat, extensive nausea, and accidental vomiting. There were 5-6 bouts of relatively pasty diarrhea per day. He would cry but not tear. After sleeping there was a crying sound in his throat (not a phlegmatic sound, but one due to incomplete formation of the laryngeal cartilage). He would sometimes sigh deeply, his throat was red, and sores were visible on the mucous membranes of his lower lips. His tongue was red and tending to dryness with little coat, while his pulse was soft. He perspired profusely and his sleep was restless. The cause was considered to be related to rickets with the involvement of a fungal infection. As there was damage to the qi and yin, administration of raw Fructus Crataegi was discontinued.

Margarita (*Zhen Zhu*) 30g

calcined Concha Ostreae (*Mu Li*) 15g
calcined Os Draconis (*Long Gu*) 15g
Magnetitum (*Ci Shi*) 30g
Rhizoma Coptidis Chinensis (*Huang Lian*) 1.5g
Semen Citri (*Ju He*) 4.5g

2 *ji*[3] were administered.

Third visit: August 4. The diarrhea had not abated. There was post prandial borborygmus followed by diarrhea which was yellow in color and predominantly watery, occurring 15-16 times the previous day. There was copious perspiration, inhalation was depressed, and there was still a sound in his throat. The tongue was shiny red with a slight coat and the pulse was fine and soft. The longstanding diarrhea had injured the spleen, thus measures were indicated for strengthening the spleen and benefitting the qi with the additions of securing, astringing, sour, and constraining medicinals to astringe the intestines and arrest diarrhea.

Radix Codonopsis Pilosulae (*Dang Shen*) 9g
Radix Rubrus Panacis Ginseng (*Ren Shen*) 3g
Fructus Zizyphi Jujubae (*Da Zao*) 15g
fried Fructus Terminaliae Chebulae (*He Zi*) 6g
fried Semen Myristicae Fragrantis (*Rou Guo*) 6g
Semen Papaveris (*Ye Ying Su*) 4.5g
Fructus Schizandrae Chinensis (*Wu Wei*) 3g

2 *ji*

---

3 The word *ji* literally means formula. It cannot be translated accurately as either dose, packet, day's supply, or any other term. Since translating it literally as formula seems confusing or awkward in English, we have chosen to leave it in Chinese *pinyin*.

Fourth visit: August 6. The diarrhea clearly diminished following administration of the medication and [the stools] had become formed. Twice the previous day he had had copious urination and his abdominal distension had gradually diminished, although some borborygmus remained. He was in good spirits and the oral erosions had ceased. His tongue tip was red with no coat and the pulse was fine and soft. Four more doses of the original prescription were administered.

Fifth visit: August 12. The diarrhea had ceased and there were 1-2 bowel movements daily. The patient's appetite had improved, as had his spirits, and the medicine had been discontinued for two days, whereupon the bowel movements increased to 7-8 times a day, becoming sticky and yellow. The spleen vacuity had not been resolved and the original prescription was administered again for another week.

Sixth visit: August 19. The diarrhea had ceased. He perspired profusely, however, and suffered from fright and restlessness upon waking. The tongue had a slight coat and the pulse was soggy. The plan was to strengthen the spleen, boost the qi, and secure the exterior with the use of sour astringents to restrain the yang.

Radix Codonopsis Pilosulae (*Dang Shen*) 9g
Radix Rubrus Panacis Ginseng (*Ren Shen*) 3g
Fructus Zizyphi Jujubae (*Da Zao*) 15g
fried Fructus Terminaliae Chebulae (*He Zi*) 6g
fried Semen Myristicae Fragrantis (*Rou Guo*) 6g
Haematitum (*Dai Zhe Shi*) 12g
Radix Astragali Seu Hedysari (*Huang Qi*) 9g
Rhizoma Atractylodis Macrocephalae (*Bai Zhu*) 9g
Radix Ledebouriellae Sesloidis (*Fang Feng*) 9g
Magnetitum (*Ci Shi*) 30g
calcined Concha Ostreae (*Mu Li*) 15g

calcined Os Draconis (*Long Gu*) 15g
Fructus Schizandrae Chinensis (*Wu Wei*) 3g

7 *ji*

After taking the medication for one week, his stools normalized and the situation improved. Family members continued to administer the original prescription and after three months brought the child in for outpatient examination. At that time, the child had recovered his strength, his physique had become robust, and he weighed more than 7.5 kilograms. His spirits were lively and his facial complexion was red and moist. His sweating had ceased and his appetite was good. His sighing, upper respiratory depression, and noisy respiration had all disappeared, and his elimination had normalized.

Comment: This was a case of severe infantile diarrhea. Although it occurred as a result of breast milk damage, the longstanding diarrhea nonetheless damaged the spleen, and, as it continued over a period of days, it injured the fluids. Based on the symptoms of copious perspiration, frequent belching, inability to sleep restfully at night, the sounds in the throat, depressed fontanelle, sunken eyes, a lack of lacrimation and a dry tongue, the child was diagnosed as having rickets and a fungal infection, all accompanied by a moderate degree of dehydration. In the beginning, simple measures for strengthening the spleen, augmenting the qi, and generating fluids proved ineffective. Later on, the incorporation of sour, restraining astringents medicinals to astringe the intestines and arrest diarrhea had a clear effect. With relatively long term therapy aimed at strengthening the spleen and augmenting the qi, securing the exterior and restraining the yang, the child recovered his strength and all the symptoms of rickets disappeared.

In cases of infantile diarrhea from poor digestion due to internal milk damage, either raw sliced Fructus Crataegi as a single ingredient or ***Mai An Chong Ji*** (a preparation of the two medicinals, Fructus Crataegi and Fructus Germinatus Hordei Vulgaris) will obtain a [good] result. Fructus Crataegi and Fructus Germinatus Hordei Vulgaris aid the spleen, supplement the stomach, and promote digestive function. They also disperse accumulations of oily, greasy meat, and, in cases of milk injury resulting in diarrhea, they have the effect of dispersing fat and arresting diarrhea. Attention must nevertheless be paid to diet during the treatment phase, or a positive effect will be difficult to achieve.

Gu Wen-hua [IV]

A case of persistent diarrhea

A 13 year old male.

Initial consultation: January 2, 1976. Hemorrhagic enteritis and enteroparalysis had been diagnosed at a local hospital on November 27, 1975. There was also concomitant hemolytic staphylococcal septicemia, and, following emergency treatment, the child was out of danger. [However, the child continued to suffer from] incessant diarrhea passing 1500-2000 milliliters of watery stool mixed with undigested grain daily. This was intermixed with a pasty fluid. A broad spectrum antibiotic was administered in order to sustain the therapy. However, the diarrhea remained unimproved.

The diagnosis was post-enteric malabsorption syndrome. A Chinese medical consultation was requested for the longstanding illness with a dual depletion of qi and yin. His cheekbones were sometimes flushed red, his tongue dry and red with a slight coat, while the pulse was fine, soft, and rapid. Considering the longstanding nature of the patient's diarrhea, and that each bowel movement was like the violent rush of water from a broken dam, [the condition] was obviously related to a falling of spleen qi with intestinal vacuity and insecurity. [Zhang] Zhong-jing's ***Chi Shi Zhi Yu Yu Liang Wan*** is the primary prescription for patterns of efflux desertion in the lower warmer. The malar redness and dry tongue pertained to an insufficiency of true yin and the heavy nature of ***Chi Shi Zhi Yu Yu Liang Wan*** stems the descent [of the diarrhea], while its astringency primarily eliminates the desertion. The assistants, Radix Astragali Seu Hedysari and Rhizoma Cimicifugae (*Sheng Ma*) raise the yang and boost the qi. Based on ***Er Jiao Mei Lian Wan*** from *Zheng Zhi Zhun Sheng,* the sour restraining nature of Fructus Pruni Mume arrests diarrhea and generates fluids, while Gelatinum Corii Asini (*E Jiao*) supplements yin. Considering that this produces a relatively large amount of thick fluid, Semen Dolichoris Lablabis is added to transform dampness.

Hallyositum Rubrum (*Chi Shi Zhi*) 15g
Limonitum (*Yu Yu Liang*) 15g
Radix Astragali Seu Hedysari (*Huang Qi*) 18g
Rhizoma Cimicifugae (*Sheng Ma*) 4.5g
Fructus Pruni Mume (*Wu Mei*) 4.5g
Gelatinum Corii Asini (*E Jiao*) 4.5g
Semen Dolichoris Lablabis (*Bai Bian Dou*) 18g

3 *ji*

Second visit: Following administration of the medication the bowel movements diminished to two per day, although the volume was still about 1100 milliliters and the tongue showed no change. The amounts of Fructus Mume and Gelatinum Corii Asini in the prescription were increased and Pericarpium Punicae Granati (*Shi Liu Pi*) was added to astringe the intestines.

Hallyositum Rubrum (*Chi Shi Zhi*) 15g
Limonitum (*Yu Yu Liang*) 15g
Radix Astragali Seu Hedysari (*Huang Qi*) 18g
Rhizoma Cimicifugae (*Sheng Ma*) 4.5g
Fructus Pruni Mume (*Wu Mei*) 9g
Gelatinum Corii Asini (*E Jiao*) 9g
Pericarpium Punicae Granati (*Shi Liu Pi*) 15g

3 *ji*

Third visit: January 10. The bowel movements had decreased to once daily, the volume of which was 400-500 milliliters. The pasty fluid quality had clearly diminished as well. His facial complexion had improved and his tongue body had normalized and developed a thin moss. His pulse was still fine, rapid, and soft. As the qi and yin had recovered, the dosages of the original prescription were decreased and medicinals for supplementing the spleen were added.

Hallyositum Rubrum (*Chi Shi Zhi*) 9g
Limonitum (*Yu Yu Liang*) 9g
Radix Astragali Seu Hedysari (*Huang Qi*) 9g
Rhizoma Atractylodis Macrocephalae (*Bai Zhu*) 9g
Radix Dioscoreae Oppositae (*Shan Yao*) 9g
Fructus Pruni Mume (*Wu Mei*) 9g
Gelatinum Corii Asini (*E Jiao*) 9g
Semen Dolichoris Lablabis (*Bai Bian Dou*) 9g
Pericarpium Punicae Granati (*Shi Liu Pi*) 15g

3 *ji*

Fourth visit: January 13. The stools had assumed a pasty, dry texture, and there was some nausea and abdominal distension. The tongue was on the pale side with a slimy moss, and the pulse was as above but with spirit. This all indicated a spleen vacuity and impedance of the qi dynamic, so six ingredients from ***Xiang Sha Liu Jun Zi [Tang]*** were prescribed.

Radix Codonopsis Pilosulae (*Dang Shen*) 12g
Radix Astragali Seu Hedysari (*Huang Qi*) 9g
Rhizoma Atractylodis Macrocephalae (*Bai Zhu*) 9g
Sclerotium Poriae Cocoris (*Fu Ling*) 9g
Rhizoma Pinelliae Ternatae (*Ban Xia*) 9g
Pericarpium Citri Reticulatae (*Chen Pi*) 69?g
fried Radix Saussureae Seu Vladimiriae (*Mu Xiang*) 9g
Fructus Seu Semen Amomi (*Sha Ren*) 3g
Hallyositum Rubrum (*Chi Shi Zhi*) 9g

7 *ji*

Fifth visit: January 19. The stools had become formed and, thus, the medicinals in the previous prescription were too fragrant and drying. This resulted in a slightly red tongue with a split down the middle, and a thin, yellow coat, while the pulse remained soft. Supplementation of the spleen and augmentation of the qi with nourishment of the stomach and generation of fluids was appropriate.

Radix Codonopsis Pilosulae (*Dang Shen*) 15g
Radix Astragali Seu Hedysari (*Huang Qi*) 12g
Sclerotium Poriae Cocoris (*Fu Ling*) 9g
Radix Dioscoreae Oppositae (*Shan Yao*) 12g
Herba Dendrobii (*Shi Hu*) 12g
raw Semen Dolichoris Lablabis (*Bai Bian Dou*) 12g
Semen Negrus Sojae (*Hei Dou Chi*) 30g
Pericarpium Citri Reticulatae (*Chen Pi*) 4.5g

Comment: Ming Li-zhong's ***Yi Zong Bi Du*** is loaded with nine measures for the treatment of diarrhea and is considered as a great compendium of the collected works of our virtuous ancestors. In the clinic, however, agile modifications must be made according to the degree of severity of the illness. Therapies are determined by whether the disease is in an early or late [stage], and there may be a single treatment progression or many measures may be used together. In the case above, the use of ***Chi Shi Zhi Yu Yu Liang Wan*** to stem descent, combining raising, sour, and restraining functions. From these examples the importance of clinical deductive process and the application of adroit and flexible principles is evident.

Xu Di-san [IV]

Zhou, a 2 month old male

Initial visit: May 7, 1976. Since birth, the child had suffered from daily diarrhea, which had continued for two months. The administration of Chinese and Western medicinals had been ineffective. He had 7-9 bowel movements over the course of the day and night, which were pale in color, thin, sticky, and slightly malodorous. There was borborygmus, frequent flatulence, and his abdomen was soft. He had a thin, white tongue coat and a fine pulse. The symptoms related to longstanding diarrhea and a failure of control of spleen transportation, thus it was spleen vacuity diarrhea. Treatment was aimed at boosting the qi and supplementing the spleen, harmonizing the middle and astringing the intestines.

Radix Pseudostellariae (*Tai Zi Shen*) 9g
Sclerotium Poriae Cocoris (*Fu Ling*) 9g
burnt Rhizoma Atractylodis Macrcephalae (*Bai Zhu*) 9g
Flos Dolichos (*Bian Hua*) 9g
Fructus Terminaliae Chebulae (*He Zi*) 9g
charred Endothelium Corneum Gigeriae Galli (*Ji Nei Jin*) 4.5g
Pericarpium Papaveris Somniferi (*Ying Su Ke*) 3g

3 *ji*

Second visit: May 10. The patient was having three bowel movements per day which were the color of the Chinese herbs. The stools had a pasty consistency and were slightly malodorous. He was having restless sleep, there were abundant night sweats, and the tongue and pulse were as above. The spleen vacuity and the transportation in the middle had not yet recovered, and I decided to keep him on the original [prescription].

Three *ji* of the original prescription were administered at the same dosage with Cinnabaris (*Zhu Sha*) [substituted for Poria].

After two more visits, the diarrhea was completely cured.

Comment: The *Nei Jing* states, "The spleen rules transportation and transformation, the stomach rules reception and absorption." Digestion and assimilation is completely dependent on digestive function and measures for the treatment of diarrhea are pushed mainly towards supplementation of the spleen and harmonization of the stomach. Prescriptions such as Qian Yi's *Wu Wei Yi Gong [Tang]* and *Chi Wei Bai Zhu [San]* are all based on this. Xue Qi said,

> Pressure damage to the stomach causes vomiting and damage to the spleen causes diarrhea.....if no [other] symptoms...then *Si Jun Zi Tang* may be used to good effect.

The comments of Qian and Xue should be deeply considered. In the above medical record of this case over the previous two months, the longstanding diarrhea had damaged the spleen, causing a loss of control over splenic transportation and difficult digestion of the breast milk. The color of the stool was, therefore, relatively bland and it was thin, sticky, and a little malodorous. Measures employing ***Si Jun Zi Tang*** assisted by Endothelium Corneum Gigeriae Galli and Semen Dolichoris Lablabis were adopted to harmonize and transform; while Fructus Terminaliae Chebulae and Pericarpium Papaveris Somniferi were employed to astringe the intestines with the hope of rapidly arresting the diarrhea. The illness had a rather long course and, although administration of both Chinese and Western medicinals had been ineffective, administration of 6 doses of this prescription produced a complete cure. While this prescription may seem rather insipid, when employed in the treatment of spleen vacuity diarrhea, it achieves a satisfactory result time and again.

Pericarpium Papaverus is an important medicinal in this prescription for the treatment of longstanding diarrhea. When used appropriately, it has an obvious effect. Nevertheless, morphine like medicinals have toxic components. If they are used inappropriately, they may result in unfavorable consequences. The characteristics [of this medicine] must be well understood and it must not be used indiscriminately. Our ancestors had a great deal of experience in the appropriate use this medicinal. For instance, *Ru Men Shi Xi* states:

> In the case of a sudden downpour of incessant watery diarrhea, medicinals such as Pericarpium Papaveris Somniferi (*Ying Su Ke*) may not be used. [This is because] even if the diarrhea is arrested, the qi in the stomach and intestines will become stagnant and stopped up, causing abdominal distension....

Li Gao said:

> Although [Pericarpium Papaveris Somniferi] may be victorious in treating even acute illnesses, it can nevertheless kill a man as surely as a sword, and so profound caution is indicated.

He also said:

> This contracting medicinal is for later use; the root of the illness must first be eliminated and it should not be hastily thrown in.

Zhu Zhen-ding said:

> [Pericarpium Papaveris Somniferi] is not indicated for use in the early stages, however, when the diarrhea is longstanding, the qi is dispersed and uncontracted, then it is appropriate to astringe, secure, contract and constrain it.

The book entitled *Xuan Ming Fang* notes:

> Where this is no depletion detriment of the true qi and a repletion pathogen is present, [Pericarpium Papaveris Somniferi] is contraindicated for use.

In general, it is inappropriate to use [Pericarpium Papaveris Somniferi] in the early acute stage of illness. For instance, abdominal pain (such as abdominal pain preceding diarrhea which is ameliorated following the diarrhea, or in the case of infants where the stool is often preceded by fussing and crying which calms down after the stool), tenesmus, an unusual sour odor to the stool, torpid intake, and poor absorption, a thick, slimy tongue coat, or a dirty, slimy tongue coat are indicative of a repletion pathogen pattern. None of these are appropriate symptoms. Even though [Pericarpium Papaveris Somniferi] is used, the dosage and usage must be based upon age. It is not appropriate to use excessive amounts or to administer [Pericarpium Papaveris Somniferi] for a prolonged period of time or it will be injurious and not beneficial. Pericarpium Papaveris Somniferi differs from other medicinals for astringing the intestines such as Fructus Terminaliae Chebulae and Pericarpium

Punicae Granati. Aside from being indicated for use in astringing the intestines in cases of longstanding diarrhea, Pericarpium Papaveris Somniferi is best if fresh, while if prepared it is used to arrest cough. These additional notes have been included only as food for thought.

DELIVERANCE

On the Administration of Chinese Medicinals to Children.

For practitioners of Chinese medicine, one of the most limiting factors in treating children in the West is the administration of therapies. Aside from being uneconomical, modalities such as acupuncture can present obvious difficulties in administration and compliance. The use of magnets and ion pellets are certainly useful as adjunctive therapies and are easy to administer. However it is my experience that in all but the most minor conditions, they most often fall short of being a satisfactory treatment modality by themselves. The administration of *tui-na* massage is a powerful modality if repeated regularly, but can be impractical to do three or four times a week. Due to its intrinsically energetic nature, teaching *tui-na* strokes to parents untrained in energy work frequently achieves less than ideal results as well.

Given the abundance of literature in Chinese on the herbal treatment of children, I have been drawn back time and again to herbal medicine as a potential modality for pediatric clients. Given the cornucopia of pediatric literature in Chinese, however, I have been surprised at the dearth of information on actually delivering medications to children beyond the odd prescription steamed in a peach and so on. As anyone who has ever taken a decoction can imagine, administration of Chinese herbs to children can be a nightmare. Most parents either balk at a forceful approach or simply grow weary of it altogether and gradually discontinue treatment. Chinese parents, it seems, largely just grin and bear it, confident in the knowledge that this torture is good for their child.

As for other methods of delivering medications to children, many children either refuse or have not yet learned how to take pills, which severely limits the viability of this method, especially in infants. While often easy to administer, specifically pediatric proprietary medicines in powder form such as ***Hou Tsao San*** and ***Hui Chun Tan***, tend to be expensive for extended administration in chronic conditions. For that matter, it is not so rare for a child to refuse a bottle with ***Hou Tsao San*** dissolved in it. Desiccated extracts from Meridian or Brion are often met with low compliance due to the tendency of the granules to stick in the back of throat like a mouthful of sand. While many of these methods sound nice in theory, compliance falls short in clinical practice.

The advent of Chinese herbal tinctures holds a great deal of promise and I think that their utility will increase with more sophisticated extraction techniques. As it stands now, however, it is my feeling that they fall far short of the potency of decoctions or even simply powdered bulk herbs administered in low doses in gelatin caps. Many of my adult clients have confided to me that they simply double my recommended dosages when taking tinctures, and this seriously compromises the cost effectiveness of this approach. Although the cost to dosage ratio is more reasonable in children, I have frequently found the phlegm resolving formulae in tinctures to be inadequate in resolving those deep phlegmatic respiratory conditions so common in children during the winter. Tinctures, however, do seem to be quite adequate for maintenance dosages and constitutional work.

A few years ago, having grown frustrated with my lack of success using tinctures, I resorted to prescribing a decoction for a 3 year old client with a particularly nasty case of bronchitis. Chinese babies and parents not withstanding, I had always winced at the thought of feeding a child an herbal decoction. The child's mother was desperate to keep him off of another round of antibiotics, however, and so seemed willing to do whatever it took to see her son recover. She reported back a few days later that he was much improved. When I inquired as to how she had fared in administering the medicine I was surprised to hear that there had been no problem. It seems her son had grown accustomed to the ritual of receiving tinctures via dropper and that any medication was acceptable as long as administered in this way.

Taking this ball and running with it, I have routinely prescribed decoctions for children delivered via dropper with great success and compliance ever since. The small amounts of a comparatively dilute liquid squirted into the child's mouth seems to be much more acceptable to many children than the prospect of swallowing even a few teaspoons of the same liquid in a few gulps. Even children who balk at the bitterness of tinctures largely do better on dropper decoctions, even bitter ones, probably because they are non alcoholic and generally taste milder than tinctures. Strange as it may seem, compliance via dropper is higher than any other form of delivery I have come across, even when numerous droppers are administered at a given time. It is by far the most effective method of administration I have used and it allows for the utilization of a full medicinal repertoire as well as individualized modification.

My personal preference is to decoct a prescription in 2-3 cups of water, simmer it down to 1 fairly thick cup of liquid and strain it. One cup can last up to a few weeks in infants. As the condition improves and or evolves, I often end up wanting to modify a prescription before the patient has finished with a given batch. Given the low cost of this approach, however, I will typically just write another prescription, although it is a simple matter to add an ingredient or two to the existing decoction for another 20 minute cooking. Since the issue of mold growth in bulk medicinals themselves and in decocted prescriptions is not to be taken lightly, I suggest that the parent keep only a few days worth in the dropper bottle and refrigerate the rest to prevent spoilage. Once or twice during the summer I will get a call from a client that a prescription has suddenly ceased to be effective and tastes funny to boot. This is generally because a prescription has begun to ferment.

Although Chinese pediatric texts seem to vary widely on this matter, doses of each ingredient for infants rarely exceed 3 grams and doses of 3—6 grams of the primary medicinals are typical in children up to age 12. It is not uncommon to see a classical prescription with typical adult doses used for pediatric purposes. The amount which the child actually receives at a given time is, however, often substantially reduced.

Infants receive 6—8 drops of decoction 2—6 times daily while a standard dose for a two year old tends to be 4 droppers twice daily. Older children may receive as much as 8 droppers 4—5 times daily in a severe acute condition. At that dosage, the psychological utility of dropper administration over simply drinking the same amount of a bitter brew in a cup is evident.

In most conditions I advise against sweetening the formula to make it more palatable to young taste buds. On the other hand, as a matter of practicality, if some sort of adulteration is the only way the child will take the medication, then this is better than nothing. Yin vacuity patterns, particularly those of the lungs as in some types of late stage bronchitis, are among those most amenable to sweetening. This is because the medicinals used in the prescription themselves often tend to be sweet.

Barley malt sugar is often preferable to honey if a sweetener is to be used. The sliding nature of honey makes it a poor choice for children with chronically loose stools. It should be kept in mind that honey is contraindicated in infants due to the risk of botulism. Small amounts of medicinals such as Semen Raphani (*Lei Fu Zi*) and Herba Eupatori (*Pei Lan*) may be included in the prescription to offset the tendency of barley malt to produce dampness and heat. Honey is a good sweetener in cases of constipation due to stagnant heat and yin vacuity where it's moistening and sliding qualities can enhance the effect of the prescription.

The only delivery system which seems to work for every child is homeopathic, and that is entirely another matter to be explored. In terms of traditional Chinese pediatrics I have come full circle, simply modifying the time honored method of taking medicines in a manner more palatable to Western children.

In the time since I originally wrote this essay it has become clear to me that children will simply take as much of a decoction as they will take; no more, no less. My precise prescribing with regard to dosage often goes out the window and the parent simply administers as much of the medication as possible to the child. In the vast majority of situations I will now say, "Give him or her as much as possible, your best effort." This seems to work well and takes the pressure off the parent as well.

STONE WOMB

The Chinese Medical Treatment of Infertility

Li Heng-you [VI]

Translator's note: The prescriptions referred to in the following cases by Li Heng-you are listed after the cases as this is how they appear in the original Chinese.

Two cases utilizing "[artificial menstrual] cycle I, II, III prescriptions" in the treatment of infertility.

Case 1: Li, a 28 year old married female:

Initial visit: February 5, 1979

Main complaint: The patient's menarche was at 14 years of age and her menstrual cycle was 2-8 days/30-40 days. In 1973, as a consequence of irregular vaginal bleeding, she was diagnosed via D&C as having endometriosis. Since that time, she had frequently suffered from obstructed menstruation and required progesterone injections to begin her flow again.

Diagnostic examination: She had occasional lumbar pain and a chilled sensation in her lower abdominal area. Her pulse was deep and her tongue was pale with tooth marks on the sides. Gynecological examination revealed no abnormalities other than that her uterus was a little small. D&C revealed no luteal phase. Her basal body temperature was monophasic as well (*i.e.*, revealed a lack of progesterone). The diagnosis was failure to ovulate which was the cause of the infertility.

Pattern discrimination: Vacuity of kidney yang.

Treatment measures: Following initial use of [artificial menstrual] Cycle I prescription for three menstrual cycles, the menstrual cycle normalized, the flow was moderate and not excessive, although her core temperature remained monophasic. With continued administration of Cycle I prescription for two more cycles, she discontinued the medication for two months. She was seen again in March of 1980. As she had clear chill in her lower abdomen, the discrimination was kidney vacuity and uterine cold. Treatment was to warm the kidney and uterus, so Cycle III prescription was given for one cycle. Her body temperature shifted, becoming biphasic, and she conceived. In November of 1980 she gave birth to a baby boy after a normal pregnancy.

Case 2: Zhang, a 25 year old female.

Initial visit: June 6, 1981.

Main complaints: The patient had been married more than three years and had not conceived. Menarche was at the age of 16 and her menstrual cycle was 7 days/45-90 days, with a scanty, pale red flow. In the past five months there had been obstructed menstruation. Pathological report revealed that there was excessive growth of the endometrium during the luteal phase and that the basal body temperature was monophasic (*i.e.*, there was too much progesterone).

Diagnostic examination: She had occasional lumbar soreness and premenstrual breast distension. Her pulse was fine and wiry, and her tongue had a thin, yellow coat. The cause of the infertility was diagnosed as a failure to ovulate.

Pattern discrimination: Kidney vacuity and liver depression.

Treatment measures: [Artificial menstrual] Cycle I prescription *Tu Rong He Ji* was given with the additions of Fructus Meliae Toosendanis (*Chuan Lian Zi*), Cortex Albizziae (*He Huan Pi*), and Radix Achyranthis Bidentatae (*Niu Xi*) to supplement the kidney and course the liver. Following treatment for three cycles her menstruation normalized, her temperature became biphasic, and she conceived and gave birth.

Discussion: The mechanism for the production of menses is based upon the concepts that the "kidneys store the essence", "the kidneys rule reproduction", and "the *chong* [*mai*] is the sea of blood, while the *ren* [*mai*] rules the womb and the fetus". Kidney supplementation is thus integrated in common clinical usage as the primary therapy and prescription measure, and this has a positive therapeutic effect in the treatment of menstrual disorders and infertility. In 1963, an attempt was made to discover the primary [treatment] measures for kidney supplementation in practice by means of integrated Chinese and Western medical research. [This approach] was modeled upon the physiological shifts that take place throughout the course of the menstrual cycle. Distinct medicinal substances were then used for distinct phases [within this cycle] in order to regulate the "kidney—*tian kuei*—*chong* and *ren*—uterus" continuum and bring it into balance. This achieved the intent of the words "regulate the menstruation" [*tiao jing*]. My college has repeatedly employed kidney supplementation in the clinic as a primary artificial Chinese herbal therapy. (The simplified name of this is Chinese Phase I). Quickening of the blood and transformation of stasis is [another] primary artificial Chinese herbal therapy. (The simplified name of this is Chinese Phase II). Warming the kidney and uterus is [another] primary artificial Chinese herbal therapy, (the simplified name of which is Chinese Phase III).

The kidney is the root of former heaven and the root of the original qi. It governs storage of the essence qi and helps promote the functions of growth and reproduction within the body. If there is infertility with diminished ovulatory function or incomplete uterine development, this is always due to kidney vacuity. Treatment of infertility, therefore, hinges on kidney supplementation. However, there must be a discrimination of patterns since vacuity of kidney yang, vacuity of kidney yin, as well as kidney vacuity with liver depression, kidney vacuity with stasis, and kidney vacuity with cold uterus are all distinct types [of disorders]. Clinically then, a pattern discrimination between Chinese Cycle I, II, and III must be made in order to maximize the therapeutic effect.

A failure to ovulate was diagnosed as the cause of the infertility in Cases 1 and 2. While these both pertain to the Chinese medical pattern discrimination of kidney vacuity, they are, nevertheless, distinct [patterns] and the therapies therefore differed. In Case 1 the obstructed menses, infertility for 10 years, lumbar soreness, sensation of chill in the lower abdomen, deep pulse, and pale tongue all pertained to a kidney vacuity with a cold uterus, and so treatment was to warm the kidney and uterus. Initial use of Chinese Cycle I to supplement the kidney yang normalized the menses, although there was still no ovulation. Seeing that there was an obvious sense of chill in the lower abdominal region, a statement by Fu Qing-zhu has bearing on this:

> Cold water's earth will not grow grass and wood, and the deepest yin's abyss does not produce fish and dragons, then if the uterus is cold can there be conception?

As there was a vacuity of kidney yang and a failure to warm the uterus, *chong* and *ren*, Chinese Cycle III was therefore used in the pre ovulatory and ovulatory phases to warm the kidney and uterus over five doses with the intent of achieving ovulation and conception.

In Case 2 the patient had been married three years and had not conceived. She had lumbar soreness, premenstrual breast distension, a fine, wiry pulse and a thin, yellow tongue moss, the pattern discrimination of which was kidney vacuity and liver depression.

Fu Qing-zhu's statement:

> Because the bosom and the uterus are habitually maligned, there is a depressive binding of liver qi and therefore this results in infertility due to envy.

Treatment [measures] were indicated to supplement the kidney and course the liver. Chinese Cycle I with the addition of Fructus Meliae Toosendanis (*Chuan Lian Zi*) and Cortex Albizziae (*He Huan Pi*) to course the liver and relieve depression and to promote ovulation and conception was used. In this sort of patient, treatment with Chinese Cycle I prescriptions should still be used as therapy, alternated with administration of formulae such as ***Xiao Yao San*** or ***Kai Yu Zhong Yu Tang*** to promote orderly reaching and soothing of liver qi. This, therefore, promotes ovulation and conception.

In the third and fourth cases, there was obstructed menstruation and a failure to conceive after many years. In the third case, diagnostic curettage confirmed the dysfunction of endometrial secretions and the pattern discrimination was that of kidney vacuity (with the tendency toward yang vacuity). Kidney supplementation and yang assistance was the indicated treatment. Chinese Cycle I was administered and the patient conceived within two cycles.

The patient in the fourth case suffered from polycystic ovaries and even following surgical techniques she was not ovulating. She had symptoms of irregular menstruation occurring at no fixed time, red or purple clotted menstrual blood, and pre-menstrual breast distension. Her pulse was deep and her tongue body was slightly dull. This fell within the category of kidney vacuity and liver depression with simultaneous blood stasis, so Chinese Cycle II was employed as the primary prescription to quicken the blood and transform stasis. This was alternated with ***Xiao Yao San*** and she then ovulated and conceived.

As a consequence of lengthy clinical experience, it is my feeling that kidney supplementation is the primary Chinese herbal therapy (Chinese [artificial menstrual] cycle I). The prescriptions and medicinals are simple and convenient and are appropriate for widespread outpatient application. [This prescription effectively treats insufficient ovulatory function giving rise to patterns of infertility such as those associated with menstrual irregularity, obstructed menstruation, menorrhagia, or scanty menstruation, failure to ovulate, or incomplete uterine development. It is also used [in the treatment of] dysfunctional uterine bleeding, and hemostasis in the post menstrual phase. ***Zu Rong He Ji*** (an empirically drafted prescription) is the primary prescription for supplementing the kidneys and promoting ovulation and is based upon the organizational principles of the mutual roots of yin and yang. [For instance] in kidney yin vacuity, in the midst of medicinals for enriching the yin, the use of medicinals such as Herba Cistanchis (*Rou Cong Rong*) and Rhizoma Curculiginis Orchoidis (*Xian Mao*) are indicated to warm and supplement the kidney, as this enriches the yin without being greasy.

In kidney yang vacuity, in the midst of medicinals for supplementing the yang, medicinals such as Radix Coquitus Rehmanniae (*Shu Di*) and Radix Dioscoreae Oppositae (*Shan Yao*) are indicated as this warms the yang without being overly drying. Yin and yang have a mutual root, and, if they mutually enrich and generate one another, a balance of yin and yang is achieved. Furthermore, Rhizoma Curculiginis Orchoidis (*Xian Mao*) functions within the prescription to excite the nerves. Based upon evidence gleaned from clinical practice, the use of this prescription promotes follicle maturation and ovulation in the pre-ovulatory phase, is effective in addressing non ovulatory menstruation and luteal dysfunction, and is useful in promoting growth in cases of incomplete uterine development.

I used Chinese Cycle I prescription in the initial treatment of a patient with polycystic ovaries who, upon examination, showed continuously elevated hormonal levels. A pasty, congealed fluid flowed continuously from her cervix, which would crystalize after leaving the body. Her body temperature was monophasic and so she was unable to menstruate. As a result of this, I felt that supplementation of the kidney with Chinese [artificial menstrual] cycle therapy was indicated to increase hormonal levels and promote follicle maturation. Nonetheless, I was unable to initiate ovulation in the polycystic ovary/ies. Since the enveloping superficial membrane layer is often excessively thick in polycystic ovaries, the ovum may mature but cannot be expelled. This means that, in general, ovulatory function and failure to ovulate have different [patterns and treatments]. From the Western medical perspective, treatment of this illness requires wedge resection[1] to disinhibit ovulation. I realized that in Chinese medicine, prescription measures for purgation and supplementation were required for the treatment of this disease. In the pre-ovulatory phase, ***Tao Hong Si Wu Tang*** in modified form was administered to quicken the blood and transform stasis, thereby the intent of ovulation was achieved. As a result of this, quickening the blood and transforming stasis was a primary focus in

---

1 This technique is no longer used. It involved the removal of a wedge from the ovary to allow the expulsion of ovum and was rarely successful.

Chinese artificial cycle therapy (Chinese Cycle prescription II). Between 1963 and 1964, the ward of integrated Chinese and Western medicine at my college used Chinese Cycle prescription II formulae in the treatment of four cases of patients with polycystic ovaries with the intent of promoting ovulation. Three of the women conceived and gave birth. Whenever infertility pertains to a pattern of kidney vacuity and stasis, such as in the case of the polycystic ovaries, or with evidence of concurrent blood stasis, Chinese Cycle prescription II is indicated for treatment.

Appendix: Chinese Herbal [Artificial Menstrual] Cycle Therapy

1. Supplementation of the kidneys as a primary Chinese herbal artificial menstrual cycle therapy (simply referred to as Chinese Cycle I)

Phase	Therapeutic Function	Prescription
Post-menstrual (days 6-10 of cycle)	Supplement *chong* & *ren* to assist ovulatory function	*Wu Ya Tiao Jing Wan*, 1 pill twice daily *Tai Pan Pian*, 5 slices, twice daily
Pre-ovulatory & ovulatory (days 11—16)	Supplement kidney to promote follicular development in ovulation	*Zu Rong He Ji*: See ingredients listed below
Premenstrual to menstrual (3—5 days premenstrually through menstruation)	Quicken blood & regulate menses to promote arrival of menstruation	*Tiao Jing Huo Xue He Ji*: See ingredients listed below

Prescriptions:

Zu Rong He Ji: Semen Cuscutae (*Tu Si Zi*) 12g, Radix Dioscoreae Oppositae (*Shan Yao*) 12g, and Radix Coquitus Rehmanniae (*Shu Di*) 12g, Fructus Lycii Chinensis (*Gou Qi Zi*) 10g, Radix Dipsaci (*Xu Duan*) 10g, and Radix Angelicae Sinensis (*Dang Gui*) 10g, Rhizoma Cyperi Rotundi (*Xiang Fu*) 6g, Herba Cistanchis (*Rou Cong Rong*) 6g, Herba Epimedii (*Xian Ling Pi*) 6-10g.

With a tendency toward yin vacuity, add Fructus Ligustri Lucidi (*Nu Zhen Zi*) 10g, and Herba Ecliptae Prostratae (*Han Lian Cao*) 12g. With a tendency toward yang vacuity, add Cornu Cervi Degelatinum (*Lu Jiao Shuang*) and Folium Artemesiae Argyii (*Ai Ye*).

Tiao Jing Huo Xue He Ji: Radix Angelicae Sinensis (*Dang Gui*) 12g, Semen Cuscutae (*Tu Si Zi*) 12g, Radix Rubrus Paeoniae Lactiflorae (*Chi Shao*) 10g, Herba Lycopi Lucidi (*Ze Lan*) 10g, and Sclerotium Poriae Cocoris (*Fu Ling*) 10g, Rhizoma Ligustici Wallichii (*Chuan Xiong*) 6g, Rhizoma Cyperi Rotundi (*Xiang Fu*) 6g. If there is extreme abdominal pain, add Rhizoma Corydalis Yanhusuo (*Yuan Hu*) 6-10g, fresh and fried Feces Trogopterori Seu Pteromi (*Wu Ling Zhi*) 5g each. In treating infertility, these medicinals are not to be administered premenstrually. Once the menses has begun they may be administered[2]. With a tendency

---

2 The use of blood quickening medicinals in treating infertility is a delicate business. While blood stasis must be eliminated, it is imperative that one not induce a miscarriage by overly coursing the blood, especially in the premenstrual phase. Physicians will often counsel their patients to avoid trying to become pregnant for a number of cycles while they administer blood quickening medicinals, hence the note to avoid administering them premenstrually.

toward vacuity cold, ***Wen Jing Tang*** may be administered during menstruation to warm the menses and aid in fertility.

2. Quickening the blood and transforming stasis as a primary Chinese herbal [artificial menstrual] cycle therapy (simply referred to as Chinese Cycle II)

Phase	**Therapeutic Function**	**Prescription**
Post-menstrual (days 6—10)	Supplement kidneys & nourish *chong* & *ren* to promote follicular development & promote ovulation	*Cu Luan Bao Tang*: See ingredients listed below
Pre-ovulatory & ovulatory (days 11—16)	Quicken blood & transform stasis to promote maturation & ejection of ovum	*Pai Luan Tang*: See ingredients listed below
Post-ovulation (days 17—25)	Regulate liver & kidney, nourish *chong* & *ren* to strengthen corpus luteum and create favorable conditions for ovum to be embedded	*Ci Huang Di Tang*: See ingredients listed below
Premenstrual (days 25-28)	Quicken blood & regulate menses to promote expulsion of necrotic endometrium & onset of menstruation	*Tiao Jing Huo Xue He Ji* See ingredients listed below

Prescriptions:

Cu Luan Bao Tang: Radix Dioscoreae Oppositae (*Shan Yao*) 15g, Radix Coquitus Rehmanniae (*Shu Di*) 12g, Radix Polygoni Multiflori (*He Shou Wu*) 12g, Semen Cuscutae (*Tu Si Zi*) 12g, Radix Angelicae Sinensis (*Dang Gui*) 10g, Herba Cistanchis (*Rou Cong Rong*) 10g. With a tendency toward yang vacuity, add Rhizoma Curculiginis Orchoidis (*Xian Mao*) and Herba Epimedii (*Xian Ling Pi*), and with a tendency toward yin vacuity, add Fructus Ligustri Lucidi (*Nu Zhen Zi*) 12g. Five doses are administered.

Pai Luan Tang: Radix Angelicae Sinensis (*Dang Gui*) 10g, Radix Rubrus Paeoniae Lactiflorae (*Chi Shao*) 10g, Herba Lycopi Lucidi (*Ze Lan*) 10g, Radix Coquitus Rehmanniae (*Shu Di*) 12g, Rhizoma Ligustici Wallichi (*Chuan Xiong*) 6g, Semen Pruni Persicae (*Tao Ren*) 6g, Flos Carthami Tinctorii (*Hong Hua*) 6g, and Rhizoma Cyperi Rotundi (*Xiang Fu*) 6g. If there is a tendency toward yang vacuity, add Ramulus Cinnamomi (*Gui Zhi*) 6g, Caulis Milletiae Seu Spatholobi (*Ji Xue Teng*) 10g, and, if there is a tendency toward yin vacuity, then add Radix Salviae Miltorrhizae (*Dan Shen*) 12g, and Fructus Lycii Chinensis (*Gou Qi Zi*) 6g. Five doses.

Ci Huang Ti Tang: Radix Dioscoreae Oppositae (*Shan Yao*) 15g, Radix Coquitus Rehmanniae (*Shu Di*) 12g, Radix Polygoni Multiflori (*He Shou Wu*) 12g, Radix Dipsaci (*Xu Duan*) 10g, Gelatinum Corii Asini (*E Jiao*) 10g, Plastrum Testudinis (*Gui Ban*) 10g, Fructus Lycii Chinensis (*Gou Qi Zi*) 10g, Herba Cistanchis (*Rou Cong Rong*) 6g. If there is a tendency toward a vacuity of yang, then add Semen Cuscutae (*Tu Si Zi*) 10g, and Radix Angelicae Sinensis (*Dang Gui*) 10g, and, if there is a tendency towards yin vacuity, then add Fructus Ligustri Lucidi (*Nu Zhen Zi*) 10g, and Radix Salviae Miltorrhizae (*Dan Shen*) 10g, and Herba Ecliptae Prostratae (*Han Lian Cao*) 12g. Five to seven doses.

Tiao Jing Huo Xue He Ji (refer to the medicinals in Cycle I) if there is a tendency toward yang vacuity, add Ramulus Cinnamomi (*Gui Zhi*) 6g, and Caulis Milletiae Seu Spatholobi (*Ji Xue Teng*) 10g. If there is a tendency toward yin vacuity, then add Radix Salviae Miltorrhizae (*Dan Shen*) 12g. In treating infertility patterns, medicinals are not to be administered premenstrually. Once the menses has started, however, they may then be administered.

3. Warming the kidneys and the uterus as a primary Chinese herbal artificial [menstrual] cycle therapy (simply referred to as Chinese Cycle III)

Phase	Therapeutic Function	Prescription
Post-menstruation (1—5 days following cessation of menstruation)	Supplement spleen & kidneys, nourish *chong* & *ren* to create conditions for ovulation	*Gui Pi Wan,* 1 pill twice daily *Tai Pan Pian*, 5 slices twice daily
Pre-ovulatory & ovulatory (days 11—16)	Warming kidney & uterus to promote ovulation	*Wen Shen Nuang Gong He Ji*: See ingredients listed below
Premenstrual & Menstrual (3—5 days premenstrually through menstruation)	Quicken blood & regulate menses to promote onset of menstruation	*Tiao Jing Huo Xue He Ji*: See ingredients listed below

Prescriptions:

Wen Shen Nuan Gong He Ji: Radix Coquitus Rehmanniae (*Shu Di*) 12g, and Radix Angelicae Sinensis (*Dang Gui*) 12g, Radix Albus Paeoniae Lactiflorae (*Bai Shao*) 10g, Ramus Loranthi Seu Visci (*Sang Ji Sheng*) 10g, Radix Dipsaci (*Xu Duan*) 10g, Herba Cistanchis (*Rou Cong Rong*) 10g, Rhizoma Ligustici Wallichii

(*Chuan Xiong*) 6g, Cortex Eucommiae Ulmoidis (*Du Zhong*) 6g, fried Folium Artemesiae Argyii (*Ai Ye*) 6g, Ramulus Cinnamomi (*Gui Zhi*) 6g, Radix Achyranthis Bidentatae (*Niu Xi*) 6g, Semen Alpiniae Katsumadai (*Cao Dou Kou*) 3g. Five doses.

Tiao Jing Huo Xue He Ji (refer to the medicinals in Cycle I) with the additions of Ramulus Cinnamomi (*Gui Zhi*) 6g, and Caulis Milletiae Seu Spatholobi (*Ji Xue Teng*) 12g. Medicinals are not to be administered premenstrually in treating infertility patterns. Once the menses has started, however, they may then be administered[3].

Zhang Xiao-chun [VI]

One case of regulating and rectifying the liver and spleen in the treatment of infertility.

Patient: A 39 year old female

Initial visit: March, 1963

Main complaint: The patient had been married 20 years and had not conceived. Examination of the husband revealed no illness. As a result of loss of post natal regulation, she tended to contract the flu easily with cough and expectoration. Her appetite was poor and her essence spirit was devitalized. She often suffered from abdominal pain, diarrhea, and a white vaginal discharge which would pour out like a flood at high water season.

---

[3] See preivous note.

Examination: She had a pale tongue body with a slimy, white coat and a slippery, weak pulse.

Discrimination of patterns: [This illness] is related to excessive coursing and draining on the part of the liver, a downfall of spleen dampness, longstanding illness in the kidneys, and a failure of the girdling vessel to bind.

Treatment measures: Treatment was aimed initially at harmonizing the liver and strengthening the spleen, percolating dampness and arresting leukorrhea.

Prescription:

Radix Bupleuri (*Chai Hu*) 9g
Radix Albus Paeoniae Lactiflorae (*Bai Shao*) 9g
Fructus Chaenomelis Lagenariae (*Mu Gua*) 19g
Semen Plantaginis (*Che Qian Zi*) 9g
Rhizoma Cyperi Rotundi (*Xiang Fu*) 9g
Semen Dolichoris Lablabis (*Bai Bian Dou*) 12g
Semen Euryalis Ferocis (*Qian Shi*) 12g
Semen Nelumbinis Nuciferae (*Lian Zi*) 12g
Fructus Seu Semen Amomi (*Sha Ren*) 6g
Pericarpium Citri Reticulatae (*Chen Pi*) 6g
Concha Ostreae (*Mu Li*) 12g
Fructus Crataegi (*Shan Zha*) 9g
Massa Medica Fermentata (*Shen Qu*) 9g

Second visit: After taking two doses she felt that the prescription was quite appropriate for her. Another six doses were administered. Fructus Chaenomelis Lagenariae and Rhizoma Cyperi Rotundi were deleted from the original prescription and Semen Gingkonis Bilobae (*Bai Guo*) and Radix Angelicae (*Bai Zhi*) were added for continuous administration of another four doses.

Third visit: Although she had been sterile for 20 years and had never conceived, after two months the patient experienced nausea. Though it was rather doubtful that she had conceived, her pulse was relaxed, coursed, and disinhibited. For the time being, the plan was to calm the fetus and harmonize the qi.

Prescription:

burnt Rhizoma Atractylodis Macrocephalae (*Bai Zhu*) 9g
Sclerotium Poriae Cocoris (*Fu Ling*) 9g
Radix Scutellariae Baicalensis (*Huang Qin*) 9g
Radix Albus Paeoniae Lactiflorae (*Bai Shao*) 9g
Fructus Immaturus Citri Seu Ponciri (*Zhi Shi*) 9g
Fructus Seu Semen Amomi (*Sha Ren*) 6g
Caulis Bambusae In Taeniis (*Zhu Ru*) 9g
Herba Eupatorii Fortunei (*Pei Lan*) 9g
Caulis Perillae Frutescentis (*Su Geng*) 9g
Pericarpium Citri Reticulatae (*Chen Pi*) 6g
Radix Praeparatus Glycyrrhizae (*Zhi Gan Cao*) 4.5g

She was urged to take four doses.

Fourth visit: After three months she contracted a wind cold cough and expectoration, with a cloudy [stuffy] head and lumbar pain. Based upon the pattern and the evidence found in the pulse, it seemed that indeed the unicorn pearl had secretly bound. To the coursing prescription were added measures for mildly perfusing and coursing the exterior, while simultaneously consolidating the fetus.

Prescription:

Herba Seu Flos Schizonepetae Tenuifoliae (*Jing Jie Sui*) 9g
Semen Pruni Armeniacae (*Xing Ren*) 12g
Fructus Citri Seu Ponciri (*Zhi Ke*) 9g

Ramus Loranthi Seu Visci (*Sang Ji Sheng*) 9g
Rhizoma Atractylodis Macrocephalae (*Bai Zhu*) 9g
Sclerotium Poriae Cocoris (*Fu Ling*) 9g
Pericarpium Citri Reticulatae (*Chen Pi*) 4.5g
Radix Praeparatus Glycyrrhizae (*Zhi Gan Cao*) 4.5g

After two doses things calmed down and two months later when pregnancy was already more than five months along, she felt fetal movement in her abdomen. A subsequent obstetric examination confirmed that there was a fetus. The patient was extremely pleased and following a normal period of gestation and a normal labor she delivered a baby boy.

Commentary: Chen Xiu-yuan in *Fu Ke Yao Zhi* states,

> Failure to conceive in women is always due to a lack of regulation within the menstrual flow. If the menstrual flow is regulated, the body is not sick, and there is still no conception, it may be that the person is too fat and the uterus is too corpulent to receive the essence. Or it may be that the person is too emaciated such that the uterus had no blood and the essence cannot accumulate.

Clinical infertility is due mainly to unregulated menses, thus regulation of the menstruation treats infertility. Beyond this, infertility is due mainly to an abundance or depletion of the yin, yang, qi, or blood. There are no fixed treatment measures to be followed, rather one is completely reliant upon a discrimination of patterns. In this case, the lack of regulation between the liver and spleen was fairly typical and the choice of medicinals for the treatment was a common prescription for regulating the liver and spleen. The unexpected resolution of a 20-year concern also serves to show the superiority of a Chinese medical approach to treatment.

Han Bai-ling [VI]

Discrimination of patterns in two cases of infertility.

Case 1: Da Shi, 40 year old married Japanese specialist

Initial visit: Summer, 1976

Main complaint: The patient had been married 20 years and still had not conceived. The husband and wife had both undergone extensive fertility testing. Other than that the wife's uterus was slightly retroflexed, pathological changes had already been ruled out. Nonetheless, she had been treated [unsuccessfully] by many well known gynecologists in Japan and the People's Republic of China who had found nothing unusual. Now, being rather anxious to have a child, and seeking to avail themselves of the extraordinary powers of Chinese medicine, husband and wife consulted me regarding their long cherished wish.

Diagnostic examination: Her body appeared rather insubstantial. Her facial complexion was dull and stagnant looking and her spirit was depressed and restrained. Her tongue moss was slightly yellow. When asked, she reported being rash, impatient, and irascible. She had painful, swollen breasts during her menstrual period. Her periods came on time, although the blood volume was scanty with purple-black clots. She had hiccups and constipation and a dry, burning sensation in the hands and feet. Her pulse was wiry, rough, and strong.

Discrimination of patterns: Based upon the four examinations, the pattern pertained to infertility due to liver depression and qi stasis, a loss of normal coursing and draining, and obstruction in the uterine vessels [*bao mai*], resulting in an incapacity of the essence to accumulate and so conceive.

Treatment measures: Treatment measures were to course the liver and relieve depression, rectify the blood and regulate the menses via the use of modified ***Bai Ling Tiao Gan Tang.***

Prescription:

Radix Angelicae Sinensis (*Dang Gui*) 15g
Radix Rubrus Paeoniae Lactiflorae (*Chi Shao*) 15g
Radix Achyranthis Bidentatae (*Niu Xi*) 15g
Rhizoma Ligustici Wallichii (*Chuan Xiong*) 15g
Semen Vaccariae Segetalis (*Wang Bu Liu Xing*) 15g
Medulla Tetrapanacis Papyriferi (*Tong Cao*) 15g
Fructus Meliae Toosendanis (*Chuan Lian Zi*) 15g
Fructus Trichosanthis Kirlowii (*Gua Lou*) 15g
Radix Salviae Miltorrhizae (*Dan Shen*) 15g
Rhizoma Cyperi Rotundi (*Xiang Fu*) 15g
Spina Gleditsiae Chinensis (*Jiao Ci*) 5g

Three doses decocted in water.

Second visit: Having taken three doses of the medication, she experienced a loss of appetite, fatigue, and a loss of strength. Rhizoma Atractylodis Macrocephalae 15g and Radix Dioscoreae Oppositae 15g were added as well [to the above prescription] to strengthen the middle and replete the spleen.

Third visit: Having taken another three doses of the medication, all of the symptoms had diminished slightly, her appetite returned and her breast distension diminished. She was, however, experiencing lumbar pain. Thereupon, Fructus Trichosanthis Kirlowii (*Gua Lou*) and Spina Gleditsiae (*Zao Jiao Ci*) were deleted from the original prescription and 15g of Radix Dipsaci and Ramus Loranthi Seu Visci were added. The patient was urged to take the prescription long term.

In 1977 Mr. and Mrs. Da Shi had to return to Beijing as their tenure at the Heilongjiang college had expired. In the Spring of the same year she delivered a baby girl which she named Da Shi-hua, borrowing the ideogram *hua* [flower] from the Song-hua river, expressing wishes for a longstanding and well established friendship between China and Japan.

Case 2: A 28 year old married female

Main complaint: The patient had not conceived after having been married for more than three years.

Diagnostic examination: [Mrs. Zhao] was examined and no pathology was discovered. When asked about her spouse she reported that he was healthy. When asked about her menses she responded that she had experienced menarche at age 18 and that she had had a menstrual period every three to six months up to the present. Her pulse was wiry, fine, and rapid, and both *chi* positions were deep.

Pattern discrimination: After careful consideration [it was determined that] the pattern pertained to kidney vacuity infertility and treatment was aimed at former heaven and undoubtedly supplementation.

Treatment measures: A prescription for supplementing the kidney and replenishing the essence was indicated.

Prescription:

Radix Coquitus Rehmanniae (*Shu Di*) 20g
Fructus Corni Officinalis (*Shan Yu Rou*) 20g
Fructus Lycii Chinensis (*Gou Qi Zi*) 15g
Radix Dioscoreae Oppositae (*Shan Yao*) 15g
Semen Cuscutae (*Tu Si Zi*) 15g

Radix Paeoniae Lactiflorae (*Bai Shao*) 20g
Cortex Eucommiae (*Du Zhong*) 20g
Radix Dipsaci (*Xu Duan*) 20g
Ramus Loranthi (*Sang Ji Sheng*) 20g
Carapax Amydae (*Bie Jia*) 15g
Plastrum Testudinis (*Gui Ban*) 20g

This was decocted in water, one prescription administered daily, with continuous administration for two months.

Mrs. Zhao reported that after obtaining an administrative position, she had returned to her hometown. Although she had not even taken the medication for two months, Mrs. Zhao became pregnant, giving birth to a baby boy after a normal pregnancy.

Comment: In the Chinese medical treatment of infertility patterns, the regulation of the menstruation is of focal importance, specifically via measures for regulation of the liver, supplementation of the kidney, transformation of phlegm, and, according to Wang Qing-ren, the expulsion of stasis. Liver depression and kidney vacuity resulting in female infertility are the most commonly observed clinical patterns. The kidney is the basis of former heaven and the root of the original qi involving reproduction; the liver controls the sea of blood by coursing and draining. In banking up, storing and securing [the blood], and when draining and coursing, the uterus stores and overflows normally. The menses are in phase, the essence is accumulated, and there is conception. If there is an insufficiency of former heaven, fatigue due to sexual excess, thwarted desires or emotional restraint, then kidney vacuity and liver depression easily result, which in turn may easily result in infertility. If [the patient] has had any abortions or has suffered from habitual miscarriage followed by infertility, these punish the kidney and treatment cannot be mistaken.

The first of these two infertility cases was due to liver depression and treatment was based on ***Bai Ling Tiao Gan Tang***. In this prescription Radix Paeoniae Rubrae, Radix Angelicae Sinensis and Rhizoma Ligustici Wallichii quicken the blood and regulate the menses, eliminate the old and generate the new. Fructus Meliae Toosendan, Fructus Trichosanthes, Radix Salvia Miltorrhizae (*Dan Shen*), and Rhizoma Cyperi course the liver and resolve depression, rectify the qi and regulate the menses. Semen Vaccariae, Medullae Tetrapanacis Papyriferi, and Spina Gleditsiae unblock [the flow of qi] in the breasts above and extend to the uterus below, and so are important medicinals for unblocking depression and dissipating bondage. In the case of infertility due to kidney vacuity, the prescription to use is ***Bai Ling Yu Yin Zhi Beng Tang*** with the deletion of medicinals which promote the resolution of congestion and the addition of Carapax Amydae, Plastrum Testudinis, Semen Cuscutae, and Fructus Lycii Chinensis for major supplementation of the true yin.

Ha Li-tian: Discrimination of patterns in three cases of infertility

Case 1: Yu, a 29 year old married female.

Initial diagnosis: April 10, 1972

Main complaint: After having been been married for four years the patient had not become pregnant. Her menses came late with a small volume and pale color and contained clots. She suffered from premenstrual distension in both breasts, lumbar soreness, and chilling lower abdominal pain. She habitually ate little and had thin stools, and her urination was clear and copious. Her four extremities lacked warmth, she had an aversion to cold in her lower limbs, and her body was fatigued and lacking strength. She suffered from a large amount of white leukorrhea, a thin body, a drawing pain in the lower abdomen, and soreness and pain in her joints.

Diagnostic examination: A gynecological examination revealed a mild cervical dysplasia, a slightly undersized uterus, and clear fallopian tubes. Her basal body temperature was recorded for two consecutive months and was monophasic. Examination via premenstrual dilation and curettage revealed endometrial hyperplasia. The diagnosis was "non ovulatory menstruation" and "primary infertility".

Pattern discrimination: The pattern pertained to a vacuity of spleen and kidney yang, cold and damp hindering the uterus, and liver depression and blood stasis.

Treatment measures: The plan was to employ measures for warming and supplementing the spleen and kidneys, dispersing cold and unblocking the collaterals.

Prescription:

Rhizoma Ciboti Barometz (*Gou Ji*) (hairs removed) 15g
Ramus Loranthi (*Sang Ji Sheng*) 15g
baked Radix Astragali (*Huang Qi*) 15g
Rhizoma Curculiginis Orchoidis (*Xian Mao*) 15g
Radix Morindae Officinalis (*Ba Ji Tian*) 15g
Sclerotium Poria Cocoris (*Fu Ling*) 12g
Herba Epimedii (*Yin Yang Huo*) 12g
fried Rhizoma Atractylodes Macrocephalae (*Bai Zhu*) 9g
Cortex Erythrinae Variegatae (*Hai Tong Pi*) 12g
Radix Clematidis Chinensis (*Wei Ling Xian*) 9g
Radix Rubiae Cordifoliae (*Qian Cao Gen*) 9g
Rhizoma Cyperi (*Xiang Fu*) 9g
Cortex Cinnamomi (*Rou Gui Yu*) 4.5g

5 *ji*[4]

This prescription was supplemented with a modification of ***Nuan Gong Wan***, one pill of which was administered daily.

Second visit: April 18th. Following administration of the medication the lumbar pain and joint pain diminished, her leukorrhea diminished, and her appetite improved. She suffered from lateral abdominal distension and pain, however, her stools were still not solid, she had gastric pain, and there was accidental vomiting and nausea. The previous measures were maintained and concurrent measures for harmonizing the stomach, nourishing the blood, and unblocking the channels were administered.

Herba Epimedii (*Xian Ling Pi*) 12g
Fructus Rubi (*Fu Pen Zi*) 12g
Folium Leptodermis Pilosa (*Mao Ye Ding Xiang Ye*) 12g
Angelicae Sinensis (*Dang Gui*) 15g
Radix Coquitus Rehmanniae (*Shu Di*) 12g
Radix Pseudostellariae (*Tai Zi Shen*) 15g
fried Rhizoma Atractylodes Macrocephalae (*Bai Zhu*) 9g
Rhizoma Pinelliae (*Ban Xia*) 9g (unprocessed)
Rhizoma Curculiginis Orchoidis (*Xian Mao*) 9g
Rhizoma Cyperi (*Xiang Fu*) 9g (powdered)
Pericarpium Citri Reticulatae (*Chen Pi*) 6g
Radix Angelicae Anomalae (*Liu Ji Nu*) 12g
Lignum Sappan (*Su Mu*) 6g

5 *ji*

4 The word *ji* literally means formula. It cannot be translated accurately as either dose, packet, day's supply, or any other term. Since translating it literally as formula seems confusing or awkward in English, we have chosen to leave it in Chinese *pinyin*.

Third visit: April 26th. Her menses began that day, [although] the volume was small and the blood was pale red. There was lumbar soreness and abdominal pain and thin runny stools which occurred 1—2 times a day. This was indicative of the failure of the descending flow of menstrual blood to enrich liver water, with concurrent insult to spleen earth. The treatment plan then was to warm and supplement the spleen and kidneys, nourish the blood and regulate the menses.

Rhizoma Cistanchis (*Rou Cong Rong*) 15g
Fructus Psoraleae Corylifoliae (*Bu Gu Zhi*) 15g
Fructus Rubi (*Fu Pen Zi*) 15g
Herba Epimedii (*Yin Yang IIuo*) 15g
Semen Cuscutae (*Tu Si Zi*) 12g
Radix Dioscoreae Oppositae (*Shan Yao*) 12g
fried Rhizoma Atractylodis Macrocephalae (*Bai Zhu*) 9g
Ramus Loranthi (*Sang Ji Sheng*) 12g
Rhizoma Cibotii (*Gou Ji*) 12g (without the tails)
Rhizoma Curculiginis Orchoidis (*Xian Mao*) 9g
Rhizoma Cyperi (*Xiang Fu*) 9g (powdered)
Herba Lycopi Lucidi (*Ze Lan*) 9g
Radix Glycyrrhizae (*Gan Cao*) 6g

4 *ji*

Fourth visit: May 2nd. [The patient's] menstruation lasted for six days and then ceased. The volume was moderate and the color was normal, although there were still blood clots. All the symptoms of lumbar soreness and abdominal pain were less than she had previously experienced. The business of pregnancy does not conform to timetables. Therefore, the plan was to use pills to slowly regulate [the menses] and, when the menstruation had normalized, conception would occur. Ten pills each of ***Jin Gui Shen Qi Wan*** and ***De Sheng Dan*** were administered morning and afternoon respectively with boiled water.

Fifth visit: May 20th. Today the patient experienced lumbar soreness and abdominal sagging, urgent lateral abdominal pain, and slight bilateral breast distension. This was evidence of her [body's] desire to begin menstruation. Her pulse was wiry and slippery and her tongue was pale red. The plan was to supplement the kidney and nourish the blood, rectify the qi and regulate the menses. This was assisted by benefiting the qi a little, in order to add force in guiding the flow.

Prescription:

Ramus Loranthi (*Sang Ji Sheng*) 15g
Rhizoma Cibotii (*Gou Ji*) (without tails) 15g
Radix Dipsaci (*Xu Duan*) 12g
Rhizoma Cistanchis (*Rou Cong Rong*) 12g
Radix Angelicae Sinensis (*Dang Gui*) 9g
Radix Paeoniae Lactiflorae (*Bai Shao*) 9g
Radix Codonopsis Pilosulae (*Dang Shen*) 12g (wild)
Rhizoma Cyperi (*Xiang Fu*) 9g (powdered) 9g
Fructus Citri Seu Ponciri Immaturus (*Zhi Ke*) 4.5g
Rhizoma Sparganii (*Sang Leng*) 9g
Rhizoma Zedoariae (*E Zhu*) 9g
Squama Mantidis Pentadactylae (*Chuan Shan Jia*) 4.5g
Resina Myrrhae (*Mo Yao*) 4.5g
Gummum Olibani (*Ru Xiang*) 4.5g

6 *ji*

Four of the above formulae were administered, and then the patient's menses began. This time she had had a 28 day cycle and the color and volume of her flow was normal. Following her menses the same medicinals as before were administered in pill form [*i.e.*, ten pills each of ***Jin Gui Shen Qi Wan*** and ***De Sheng Dan*** administered morning and afternoon with boiled water]. During subsequent menstrual phases 3—5 *ji* of the prescription from the fifth visit were administered. She recuperated for many months, and her basal body temperature again became biphasic. On a return visit on Feburary 13th, 1973 she had already missed five menstrual periods, she had a bland tasteless sensation in her mouth, and she craved sour and detested oils. These were good signs that she had conceived. A pregnancy test was administered which was indeed positive, so a prescription was written to benefit the kidneys and protect the fetus, rectify the qi and harmonize the stomach. She did this therapy for more than a month and then the medicinals were discontinued. In July of 1973 she gave birth and both mother and child were well.

Comment: In this case the Western diagnosis of non-ovulatory menstruation and primary infertility pertained to the patterns of a vacuity of spleen and kidney yang, insufficient transformation of the source and cold congealing in the uterus and channels. Therefore, the symptoms are scanty, pale menstruation, lumbar soreness, abdominal pain, chilled limbs and an aversion to cold, clear, thin, white leukorrhea, pasty stools and clear urine. Rhizoma Cibotii, Rhizoma Curculiginis, Herba Epimedii, Rhizoma Cistanchis, Fructus Rubi, and Cortex Cinnamomi warmed the kidneys, dispersed cold, and supplemented the true essence of the kidney; Radix Angelicae Sinensis, Radix Paeoniae Lactiflorae, Ramus Loranthi, Radix Coquitus Rehmanniae, and Folium Leptodermis Pilosae enrich and supplement the liver and kidney, nourish the blood, and regulate the channels; Radix Codonopsis, Radix Astragali Seu Hedysari, Rhizoma Atractylodis Macrocephalae, Sclerotium Poria Cocoris, and Radix Dioscoreae Oppositae fortify the spleen and benefit the qi, in order to enrich and transform the source. Once the kidney yang is warmed and the essence and blood are nourished, then the uterus becomes strong and the *chong* and *ren* are abundant. Once spleen transportation is fortified, then the qi and blood become full by themselves, and the sea of blood brims over. Simultaneous use of Radix Bupleuri, Rhizoma Cyperi, Radix Angelicae Anomalae (*Liu Ji Nu*), and

Herba Lycopi rectify the qi and quicken the blood, course and disinhibit the channels and vessels, and when the qi and blood circulate smoothly, then the menses are regulated of their own accord. The post-menstrual phase formula in decoction supplemented the spleen and kidney and harmonized the qi and blood, supplementing while simultaneously coursing. At the same time, the formula administered in pill form warmed the kidney yang and regulated the menstrual blood; in the midst of generation is transformation. Once the *chong* and *ren* are unblocked and abundant, the menses normalize, and conception is certainly possible.

Case 2: Wang, a 32 year old married female.

Initial diagnosis: July 13, 1972

Initial complaint: [The patient] had been married for seven years and had remained infertile up to the present. She habitually experienced extended menstruation of moderate amount and dark color, which typically contained clots. She suffered from premenstrual breast distension, visual dizziness and nausea, and her last menses was on June 24th, 1972. Examination revealed lateral abdominal distension and pain which did not like pressure. She had a yellowish leukorrhea which was pasty, turbid, and foul smelling, headache, costal distension, and low fever. Her Western diagnosis was "essential infertility", and "bilateral adhesions of the fallopian tubes".

Diagnostic examination: Her pulse was deep and wiry and her tongue was dark with a yellow, slimy coat.

Pattern discrimination: The pattern pertained to a stasis of qi and blood, and a binding accumulation of dampness and heat.

Treatment measures: The plan was treatment via rectification of the qi and transformation of stasis, clearing and resolving damp toxins.

Prescription:

Radix Bupleuri (*Chai Hu*) 6g
powdered Rhizoma Cyperi (*Xiang Fu*) 9g
Tuber Curcumae (*Yu Jin*) 4.5g
Radix Angelicae Dahuricae (*Bai Zhi*) 4.5g
Caulis, Calyx, and Folium Perillae (*Zi Su*) 4.5g
Radix Salviae Miltiorrhizae (*Dan Shen*) 15g
Rhizoma Sparganii (*San Leng*) 9g
Rhizoma Zedoariae (*E Zhu*) 9g
Radix Paeoniae Rubrae (*Chi Shao*) 9g
Resina Myrrhae (*Mo Yao*) 2g
Gummum Olibani (*Ru Xiang*) 2g
Squama Mantidis Pentadactylae (*Chuan Shan Jia*) 6g
Rhizoma Desiccata Polygoni Cuspidati (*Hu Chang*) 9g
Herba Cum Radice Baijiangcao (*Bai Jiang Cao*) 15g
Bulbus Shancigu (*Shan Ci Gu*) 12g

5 *ji*

Second visit: July 19th. After administration of the medication, the costal and abdominal pain and distension had slightly diminished, the leukorrhea had lessened, and the headache and nausea had been eliminated. As a healing dynamic had already been realized, the original measures were continued. The Perillae and Bulbus Shangcigu were deleted from the original prescription and 9g each of Radix Angelicae Sinensis and Concha Arcae Inflatae (*Wa Leng Zi*) were added to another six prescriptions.

Following administration of this medication, her period arrived and finished on time, and was normal color and volume as well. The blood clots diminished and there was no longer any premenstrual breast distension or abdominal pain. The plan was then to administer the medication in pill form to [consolidate] recuperation. One pill each of ***Xiao Jin Dan, Xiao Yao Wan,*** and ***De Sheng Wan*** was administered with water, morning, noon, and evening for 20 consecutive days. This was combined with 3-6 formulae of the herbal prescription from the second visit, which was administered in the last week prior to menstruation. Following menstruation the above mentioned pills were then administered. Having recuperated for ten months [with the above medications], a gynecological examination showed "unobstructed fallopian tubes" and subsequent to this she conceived.

Comment: In this case the prolonged menstruation, purple blood clots, premenstrual breast distension, and urgent lateral abdominal pain were indicative of qi stasis, and stasis and obstruction in the menstrual vessels. The headache and nausea, low fever in the morning and evening, and foul smelling leukorrhea were indicative of dampness accumulating and transforming to heat. This steamed up the stomach mansion, preventing the clear yang from rising, binding the lower warmer, and resulting in a detriment to the *dai mai*. The prescription employed Radix Bupleuri, Rhizoma Cyperi, Gummi Olibanum, and Resin Myrrha to rectify the qi and arrest pain; Tuber Curcumae, Radix Salviae Miltiorrhizae, Rhizoma Sparganii, Rhizoma Zedoariae, Radix Paeoniae Rubrae, Squama Mantidis Pentadactylae, and Concha Arcae (*Wa Leng Zi*) to quicken the blood and transform stasis, and Herba Cum Radice Baijiangcao, Rhizoma Desiccata Polygonati Cuspidati, and Bulbus Shancigu (*Shan Ci Gu*) to clear heat and resolve toxins, transform dampness and arrest leukorrhea. These are assisted by Folium Perillae to rectify the qi and harmonize the middle. Radix Angelicae Dahuricae is pungent and fragrant and outthrusts the orifices. [This formula] succeeded in progressively decreasing the symptoms so that menstruation arrived as scheduled. During the second visit Radix Angelicae Sinensis and Radix Paeoniae Lactiflorae were added to nourish the blood and regulate the menses combined with the formula in pill form to slowly [treat] the root, and in the end accumulate the essence and foster conception.

Case 3: Sun, a 28 year old married female

Initial visit: May 4, 1972

Main complaint: The patient had been married three years but had not become pregnant. Her menses had been normal in the past. However, in 1968 she developed "[hyper-]thyroidism" after which her menstruation became irregular. She had undergone Western pharmaceutical therapies but had developed symptoms of palpitations, insomnia, tremors in her hands, spontaneous sweats, and vexation heat, all of which had basically resolved. Nevertheless, her menstruation had not normalized. Gynecological examination revealed retarded uterine development but no dysplasia.

Diagnostic examination: At the time of the examination her neck was enlarged and her thyroid was swollen and enlarged upon palpation. She sometimes had a sense of being suffocated, her face was flushed red, there was lumbar soreness and lack of strength, a pasty, thick leukorrhea, and delayed menstruation with a small volume of scanty, dark blood. She had not menstruated since March 23rd. Her pulse was wiry, fine and somewhat rapid, while her tongue was red with a thick, slimy coat.

Discrimination of patterns: Dampness and turbidity congealing and stagnating, binding and becoming phlegm. As the illness was of a prolonged nature the yin aspect had become depleted.

Treatment measures: The plan was to clear heat and transform phlegm, soften hardness and disperse binding, combined with measures for benefiting the kidney yin.

Prescription:

Bulbus Shancigu (*Shan Ci Gu*) 30g
Tuber Dioscoreae Bulbiferae (*Huang Yao Zi*) 15g
Herba Sargassi (*Hai Zao*) 9g
Thallus Algae (*Kun Bu*) 6g
Squama Mantidis (*Chuan Shan Jia*) 9g
Ramus Photiniae (*Shi Nan Ye*) 12g
Fructus Ligustri Lucidi (*Nu Zhen Zi*) 12g
Herba Leonuri Heterophylli (*Yi Mu Cao*) 9g

The above medicinals were ground into a fine powder and 3g were taken brewed in brown sugar water.

In addition the following medicinals were put in a cloth bag, boiled in water, and administered twice daily as a sitting fumigation.

Fructus Cnidii (*She Chuang Zi*) 12g
Cortex Phellodendri (*Huang Bai*) 6g
Fructus Evodiae Rutecarpae (*Wu Zhu Yu*) 3g

Six bags of the above medicinals were administered. Two bags were administered consecutively and the medication was discontinued for a time and then resumed. Her neck was no longer enlarged and her thyroid could just barely be palpated. Her appetite and sleep markedly improved and her facial redness and lumbar soreness had also resolved. Her menstruation had changed as well. She menstruated on January 8, 1973 and again on February 10th. It was of normal color and amount and there was some slight premenstrual abdominal pain. The above medicinals were administered once daily in the morning, and in the evening a single pill of ***Ba Bao Shen Xun Dan*** was administered. She returned six months later for a return visit and reported that she was three months pregnant.

Comment: The *Nei Jing* states,

> First there is illness, and then later there is counterflow. Treat the root.

In this case the menses was initially normal. Following the hyperthyroid episode her menstruation became abnormal and when she married she was unable to conceive. Xiao Zhen-zhai states in *Nu Ke Jing Lun*:

> First there is an illness and afterward the menses become irregular, it is therefore appropriate to treat the illness, and oncc the disease has been eliminated, the menses then become regulated of their own accord.

The patient's sense of suffocation, thyroid enlargement, pasty leukorrhea, facial heat, and lumbar soreness were indicative of a mutual binding of phlegm and heat obstructing the airways and a descension of dampness and heat resulting in a detriment to the kidney yin. Bulbus Shancigu and Tuber Dioscoreae Bulbiferae were used in the prescription to resolve toxins and disperse swelling while simultaneously treating the leukorrhea. Herba Sargassi and Thallus Algae clear heat and disperse phlegm, soften hardness, and dissipate binding. Squama Mantidis cracks the blood and transforms stasis, unblocks the channels and quickens the collaterals. Ramus Photiniae, Fructus Ligustri Lucidi, and Herba Leonuri Heterophylli supplement the kidney and benefit the essence, enrich water and moisten wood. As the illness was of a longstanding nature and a rapid response was difficult to achieve, powdered formula was used with the intent of working slowly to achieve the effect of regulating the menses and promoting conception.

RISING TO THE OCCASION

Discussions and Case Histories on Impotence

The practice of *nan ke*, literally means andrology but implies male urogenital diseases in general. It is not traditionally considered a specialty in Chinese medicine in the way, for instance, that gynecology is. Men's reproductive health has, nevertheless, always been of great importance in the general scheme of Chinese cultural values. This is reflected in the variety of over-the-counter medications which address male sexual dysfunction as well as the wealth of relevant citations in the traditional medical literature. Of late the *Shanghai Journal of TCM (Shanghai Zhong Yi Yao Za Zhi)* has contained an article on *nan ke* in every issue. *Nan ke* in ancient times was the province of "the art of the bedroom" (*fang zhong shu*), and those physicians researching *fang zhong shu* were called *fang shu jia* or specialists (in the treatment of disorders pertaining to) the bedroom arts. Whether or not these physicians were themselves skilled in the bedroom arts is another matter.

In the People's Republic of China today, the study of *nan ke* has attracted a great deal of interest, and is currently considered a "hot topic". This seems quite fitting given the growing momentum of the men's movement in the West. It is with this in mind that I have included a chapter on *nan ke*, pertaining specifically to one of the most common men's complaints, impotence.

Impotence is virtually synonymous with kidney vacuity in the minds of many practitioners, a misconception which is easily reflected in poor clinical results. In my selection of case histories, I have tried to include some of the less obvious but quite common patterns causing this problem and have purposefully de-emphasized the more familiar patterns of vacuity of kidney yin and depletion of life gate fire. It has been my personal experience that patterns involving impotence and premature ejaculation due primarily to depressive liver heat and/or dampness and heat in the lower warmer are at least as common, if not more so, in younger men than purely kidney vacuity patterns. This is not to denigrate the importance of kidney related patterns in the treatment of impotence, and it is clear from the following cases and discussions that some degree of impaired kidney function is nearly always present. It is simply an issue of determining the relative importance of any given piece of the puzzle in any particular case. I have included two cases which deal specifically with premature ejaculation in this chapter as well. This is not for any lack of available material regarding impotence, but rather because impotence and premature ejaculation, although distinct illnesses in and of themselves, often occur together and share common patterns. I will say, however, that in my readings on premature ejaculation thus far, the literature has tended to favor vacuity patterns. For this reason, I have chosen two cases which deal primarily with kidney vacuity in the treatment of premature ejaculation. Be that as it may, it is prudent of be aware of the variety of patterns relevant to impotence when treating premature ejaculation.

The medical discussions on impotence that follow are of a rather unique nature in that they are structured in a question and answer format. This is a fairly common structure for modern medical writings and there is an entire genre of books which are simply entitled "100 questions on...". Precedents for this catechismal approach can be traced as far back as the dialogues of Huang Di and Qi Bo in the *Nei Jing.* The discussions here are by Wu Yin-gen et al. and are extracted from *Zhong Yi Nan Ke Bai Wen* (*One Hundred Questions in Chinese Medical Male Urology*).

The first discussion simply defines the terminology associated with the treatment of impotence. In the interest of space, I have left out an entire section of this discussion dealing with the biomechanics of impotence and penile erections in general as this information is readily available in English in any physiology text. The second discussion deals with pattern discrimination in the treatment of impotence, and the final discussion is an overview of traditional prescriptions pertinent to the treatment of impotence. It is my hope that, in the future, a more comprehensive treatment of issues pertaining to men's health will be available in English.

Discussions

What is yang wilt and why is it also called yin wilt? [IX]

Yang wilt [impotence] means that while one has normal sexual desire, one's penis is unable to achieve an erection and initiate sexual intercourse. It also pertains to the capacity of the penis to become erect but an incapacity to maintain sufficient firmness to complete sexual activity.

The types and kinds of impotence have been defined in order to discriminate the severity and development of the condition. For instance, an inability to achieve an erection and enter the vagina is called "complete impotence". Entering the vagina and then becoming spontaneously flaccid such that intercourse cannot be completed, leaving one unsatisfied and without ejaculation is called "incomplete intercourse". Another method of differentiation calls impotence characterized by an inability to have intercourse "primary impotence" (*yuan fa xing yang wei*), while difficulty in achieving an erection which appears only later on after a period of normal sexual relations is called "successive impotence" (*ji fa xing yang wei*). In any differentiation of the essential etiologies of impotence, factors involving the role of the essence spirit in achieving an erection must be discriminated from impotence of an organic nature.

The medical writers of ancient times have dealt with impotence in minute detail, although it has not been systematically classified. However, [these authors] have extensively described the degree of severity and the nature of impotence. For instance, *Ma Wang Tui Yi Shu: Tian Xia Dao Tan* delineates five types of situations [regarding impotence]: 1.) Failure to rise. [This means that] the penis cannot become erect. 2.) [The penis may become] angry (literal) but does not enlarge. This means that while the penis becomes erect, it fails to thicken. This is due to a failure of the qi and the blood to flow into the genital region. *Yi Xin Fang* offers quite an incisive description of these two conditions:

> The jade stalk does not become angry [aroused] and the qi fails to arrive, or [the penis may become] angry but does not enlarge; the qi of the flesh has not arrived.

This statement means that the penis may fail to achieve an erection due to lack of desire, or that the desires within one's heart/mind are unable to reach the yin stalk. The penis may become erect but does not thicken. This is due to a failure of the qi and blood to nourish the genital region. 3.) [The penis may be] enlarged but not firm. [This is because] the sinew qi has not arrived. The yin stalk is understood in Chinese medicine as being governed by the liver channel. The liver governs the motility of the sinew vessels and the yin stalk is the ancestral sinew. If the qi and blood cannot pour into the sinew vessels of the genital region, then the jade stalk will not harden. 4.) [The penis may] harden but not become hot. [In this case] the qi has not arrived. This description is unique to Chinese medicine and means that although the penis becomes angry [engorged], enlarged, and firm, these are merely physiological conditions and attention must still these are merely physiological conditions and attention must still be paid to one's mental state and the condition of the entire body. The failure of the qi to arrive means that the spirit qi has not arrived. Only firmness and heat [together] reflect a harmonious mind prior to sexual activity. The capacity for fulfilling and normal sexual relations is understood in Chinese medicine only in terms of the four attainments. These are the attainment of harmony, the attainment of the flesh, the attainment of the sinew, and the attainment of the qi. A lack of any one of these attainments may result in impotence. 5.) "The old do not rise." This relates to the aged and manifests as impotence due to kidney vacuity.

How are patterns discriminated in impotence? [IX]

Impotence patients most often tend to have a relatively large number of symptoms. Chinese medical theory is sufficient to discriminate as to whether the patient's pattern of illness is that of yin vacuity, yang vacuity, qi vacuity, or blood vacuity, or whether [these patterns manifest] simultaneously. The location of the illness is also easily determined and, based on the etiologies of the disease pathogens leading to impotence, the nature of these disease pathogens and their [appropriate] therapies should be discriminated as well. Nevertheless, there are patients whose only manifest symptom is impotence, having no bodily symptoms whatsoever. What then [in this case] is important to consider in terms of pattern discrimination and therapy?

1. Personal variations: Impotence in young people most commonly has three etiologies.

A. Excessive masturbation: Masturbating for relatively long periods of time or unrestrained sexual activity is called, in Chinese medicine, excessive hacking and consumption (*zhuo dai tai guo*), and this loss of essence results in impotence. This is excessive sexual stimulation and excessive taxation of the sexual organs. There is detriment damage to the kidney qi and restraint should be exercised. Therapy should not include excessive use of medicinal substances for warming the yang. Rather it is important to nourish the essence and supplement kidney yin. It is essential to use bitter tasting medicinal substances such as Cortex Phellodendri (*Huang Bo*), Rhizoma Anemarrhenae (*Zhi Mu*) and Radix Sophorae Flavescentis (*Ku Shen*) which firm up the yin [can be read as genitals] and clear fire. Turtle (*Bie Jia Yu*) should be eaten often as patients with impotence often have a yin vacuity.[1]

B. Thoughtless sexual activity with young women: This may be combined with a lack of sexual understanding, a disharmonious marriage, anger which is detrimental to the kidney qi, or poor stimulation during the course of sexual relations [*i.e.*, boring sex]. These pertain to causative factors in the realm of the emotions and innermost thoughts. When dredging these up, physicians should point out concrete situations [which may be causing problems] so that these may be understood and serve as guides [in the future]. The use of Chinese medicine should include the use of medicinals for coursing the liver and rectifying the qi or those for regulating and supplementing the heart and spleen. Some medicinals commonly used in treatment to good effect include Radix Bupleuri (*Chai Hu*), Radix Albus Paeoniae Lactiflorae (*Bai Shao*), Rhizoma Atractylodes Macrocephelae (*Bai Zhu*), Radix Angelicae Sinensis (*Dang Gui*), Herba Menthae *Bo He*), and Pericarpium Citri Reticulatae (*Chen Pi*), or ***Ren Shen Gui Pi Wan***.

---

[1] The text from which this discussion was excerpted contains two other lengthy discussions on the perils and ramifications of masturbation. While making no judgements on this matter myself, it is clearly considered a major potential detriment to sexual health in the field of andrology.

C. A weak constitution: If there is an insufficiency of [the qi of] former heaven with poor development, [a tendency toward] chronic illness, or if young people fail to get enough exercise or do very little in the way of athletics, then the quality of their physique will suffer and this also may give rise to impotence. This condition will take a relatively long time to recuperate.

Men over 45 who are impotent most often present as being overworked or there may be some concurrent, pre-existing recurrent weakness which is commonly seen as insufficiency of essence qi. The use of medicinal substances to supplement the kidney essence and supplement the kidney qi is indicated. Medicinal substances which have a bitter taste should not be employed and medicinals which nourish the yin should also not be used excessively. A depletion of yang qi is more commonly seen in men over 50 years of age, and medicinals which warm the yang and supplement the qi are appropriate. When necessary, the use of medicinals to supplement fire such as Radix Praeparatus Aconiti Carmichaeli (*Fu Zi*) and Cortex Cinnamomi (*Rou Gui*) may be appropriate. Some men who are relatively more advanced in age than their wives may find themselves unable to satisfy their wives' appetites. This will weigh heavily on a husband's mind, causing his impotence to grow progressively more severe. In this case, simply supplementing the kidney is most often to no avail. The recuperating patient must, nonetheless, diminish his sexual activity while achieving a relatively satisfying stimulus [for his wife when he does have sex]. The wives of impotence patients over 50 should be evaluated as to whether or not they are having any obvious menopausal symptoms. Changes in the mental state of these women [associated with menopause] may influence the development of impotence in the male. It is important to "work along both lines" in order to achieve a result.

Attention must be paid as to whether or not impotence in geriatric patients is due to diabetes, renal disease, coronary heart disease, arteriosclerosis, or an endocrine disorder. In these cases, impotence is only an acute symptom of a more primary illness and it is important here also to "work along both lines" in order to achieve a result.

2. Seasonal variations: In impotence due to kidney vacuity, the use of warming medicinals is indicated in the wintertime. If the impotence becomes more severe in the winter and sexual activity normalizes during the summer, the use of warming medicinals is indicated. Radix Praeparatus Aconiti Carmichaeli (*Fu Zi*), Cortex Cinnamomi (*Rou Gui*), Herba Ephedrae (*Ma Huang*), Herba Cum Radice Asari (*Xi Xin*), Rhizoma Desiccata Zingiberis (*Gan Jiang*), Cornu Cervi Parvum (*Lu Jiao*), Colla Cornu Cervi (*Lu Jiao Jiao*), Semen Alli Tuberosi (*Cong Bai*), and Fructus Foeniculi Vulgaris (*Hui Xiang*) may be selected for use and ultimately Sulphur (*Liu Huang*) (although only after it has been drug processed) may also be considered.

The excessive use of warming medicinals during the summer is not indicated. For instance, if the use of Radix Panacis Ginseng (*Ren Shen*) and Tuber Ophiopogonis Japonicae (*Mai Men Dong)* is necessary to achieve a positive result, then during the summer Radix Panacis Quinquefolii (*Xi Yang Shen*) is a better substitution.

During the course of the treatment of impotence, positive changes in the condition will first appear late at night or early in the morning (around 3-5) when some sexual excitation will be noticed, and ultimately a satisfactory erection is obtained. This is evidence of the return of the yang qi within the kidney and a timely increase in the dose of medicinal substances which supplement the kidney qi and boost the kidney yang to further consolidate the therapeutic effect is appropriate.

3. Discriminating between vacuity and repletion: Based on the observations of the ancients, vacuity patterns of impotence occur eight or nine times out of ten, and repletion patterns occur two or three times out of ten. In modern clinical experience, however, repletion pattern impotence or mixed vacuity and repletion pattern impotence is still very often seen, for instance, in cases of impotence occurring simultaneously with a turbid white flow. In this case, there is a flow of pasty, thick fluid or white, pasty, turbid fluid following a bowel movement or urination. In critical conditions, this discharge does not cease on its own, but is draining constantly. This is significant evidence of damp heat (or damp turbidity) pouring downward, and medicinal substances which clear and transform dampness and turbidity such as Cortex Phellodendri (*Huang Bo*), Herba Lophatheri Gracilis (*Zhu Ye*), Flos Lonicerae Japonicae (*Yin Hua*), Radix Lithospermi Seu Arnebiae (*Zi Cao*), Herba Cum Radice Violae (*Zu Hua Di Ding*) and Rhizoma Polygoni Cuspidati (*Hu Chang*) should be considered. Clinically, impotence is often seen occurring simultaneously with seminal emission and efflux diarrhea. This is a manifestation of an insecurity of the essence gate, and a significant etiological [factor] in insecurity of the essence gate is "a tendency to effulgence of ministerial fire" (*xiang huo pian wang*). Ministerial fire [in this case refers to] a species of fire pathogen resulting from a slight pathological tempering of an individual's bodily fluids. This may be caused by excessive worry and an unsettled spirit. Inhibited emotions with depressive binding liver qi not transforming fire may be a cause and it may also be due to wavering thoughts and desires, unfulfilled hopes, and pent up [feelings]. Clearing and draining ministerial fire are, therefore, the major therapeutic measures. Rhizoma Coptidis Chinensis (*Huang Lian*) may be combined with Gelatinum Corii Asini (*E Jiao*) to clear the heart and enrich the kidneys. Radix Bupleuri (*Chai Hu*) and Tuber Curcumae (*Yu Jin*) are combined with fried Fructus Gardeniae (*Shan Zhi Zi*) and Radix Rehmanniae (*Sheng Di*) to clear the liver and resolve depression. Radix Polygalae Tenuifoliae (*Yuan Zhi*) and Rhizoma Acori Graminei (*Shi Chang Pu*) are combined with Radix Dioscoreae Oppositae (*Shan Yao*) and Bulbus Lilii (*Bai He*) to supplement the spleen and open the orifices. These combinations of medicinal substances are all commonly used in the treatment of impotence.

In the case of impotence with blood in the semen [hematospermia] and draining seminal fluid, this is a manifestation of heat in the essence chamber and measures for cooling the blood and restraining and astringing [the blood and essence] are commonly used. Medicinal substances such as Radix Coquitus Rehmanniae (*Shu Di*), Radix Rubrus Paeoniae Lactiflorae (*Chi Shao*), Cortex Radicis Moutan (*Mu Dan Pi*), Herba Seu Radix Cephanopolis Segeti (*Da Ji*), Radix Rubiae Cordifoliae (*Qian Cao Gen*), Fructus Rosae Laevigatae (*Jin Ying Zi*), and Fructus Rubi (*Fu Pen Zi*) are commonly used in the treatment of impotence as well. In all these cases it is difficult to make a final statement. Whether or not the pattern discrimination is reliable when discussing treatment, whether or not the proper pattern has been determined before dispatching medicines, and the physician's level of theoretical and clinical understanding all have a direct and immediate relationship [to treatment outcomes]. An understanding of both common and unusual [patterns] when employed in accordance with agile utilization of Chinese medical theory can thus raise the level of therapeutic effectiveness in [the treatment of] impotence.

What are some of the essential formulae used in the treatment of impotence from dynasties past? [IX]

The prescriptions used in the treatment of impotence can be divided into six major categories listed below:

1. Prescriptions for supplementing the kidney and strengthening the yang:

Shen Qi Wan (marketed as a prepared medicine): [This prescription] was the creation of Zhang Zhong-jing of the Han Dynasty. It is composed of Radix Coquitus Rehmanniae (*Shu Di*), Radix Dioscoreae Oppositae (*Shan Yao*), Fructus Corni Officinalis (*Shan Yu Rou*), Rhizoma Alismatis (*Ze Xie*), Sclerotium Poriae Cocoris (*Fu Ling*), Cortex Radicis Moutan (*Mu Dan Pi*), Radix Praeparatus Aconiti Carmichaeli (*Fu Zi*), and Ramulus Cinnamomi (*Gui Zhi*). This prescription supplements and drains at the same time and the ingenious combination [of medicinals] achieve the intent of supplementing the kidney and boosting kidney yang. It is the model prescription for supplementing the kidney yang of that dynasty. Long term administration [of this prescription] strengthens the body, enhances immunity, and heightens excitation, thus achieving the intent of treating impotence.

You Gui Wan (available as a prepared medicine): [This prescription] was the creation of Zhang Jing-yue of the Ming Dynasty. It is ***Shen Qi Wan*** with the deletion of the three "draining medicinals", Rhizoma Alismatis (*Ze Xie*), Sclerotium Poriae Cocoris (*Fu Ling*), and Cortex Radicis Moutan (*Mu Dan Pi*), and the addition of Fructus Lycii Chinensis (*Gou Qi Zi*), Cortex Eucommiae Ulmoidis (*Du Zhong*), Semen Cuscutae (*Tu Si Zi*), Cornu Degelatinum Cervi (*Lu Jiao Shuang*), Radix Angelicae Sinensis (*Dang Gui*), and Radix Glycyrrhizae (*Gan Cao*). This prescription lays particular stress on the regulation and rectification of water and fire within the kidneys, balancing the equilibrium of the kidney yin and kidney yang. In the treatment of impotence due to a vacuity of kidney yang, it is much stronger than ***Shen Qi Wan.***

Ban Long Wan: This is composed of Colla Cornu Cervi (*Lu Jiao Jiao*), Cornu Degelatinatum Cervi (*Lu Jiao Shuang*), Semen

Cuscutae (*Tu Si Zi*), Semen Biotae Orientalis (*Bai Zi Ren*), Radix Coquitus Rehmanniae (*Shu Di*), Sclerotium Poriae Cocoris (*Fu Ling*), and Semen Psoraleae Corylifoliae (*Bu Gu Zhi*). This prescription originated in *Qing Nang Ji.* Currently however, examination of a record 550 years earlier by the author of *Yi Xue Zheng Chuan* finds the statement that a Daoist priest from Sichuan was singing a song in a drunken revelry, the words of which were:

> When the end alley cannot contain the blue sea, let alone the nine transformations of the golden elixir, only the spotted dragon's [*ban lung*] crown can prop up the pearl and supplement the flow of blood into the jade hall gate.

The spotted dragon is the deer and Cornu Cervi Parvum (*Lu Jiao*) raises the pearl. In this prescription Colla Cornu Cervi (*Lu Jiao Jiao*) and Cornu Degelatinum Cervi (*Lu Jiao Shuang*) are employed together. This name is said to have been passed down by the immortals.

2. Prescriptions for replenishing and supplementing the kidney essence:

Da Bu Yuan Jian: This is composed of Radix Panacis Ginseng (*Ren Shen*), Radix Angelicae Sinensis (*Dang Gui*), Radix Coquitus Rehmanniae (*Shu Di*), Fructus Corni Officinalis (*Shan Yu Rou*), Fructus Lycii Chinensis (*Gou Qi Zi*), and Radix Praeparatus Glycyrrhizae (*Zhi Gan Cao*). This prescription is the creation of Zhang Jing-yue of the Ming Dynasty. He states that,

> This is an important prescription for retrieving heavenly assistance, transforming and salvaging the root, and shoring up the source.

It is the ancient prescription for supplementing the kidney essence.

Da Zao Gu Zhen Wan: This is the prescription of Lin Pei-qin of the Qing Dynasty. It is composed of Radix Coquitus Rehmanniae (*Shu Di*), Radix Dioscoreae Oppositae (*Shan Yao*), Fructus Corni Officinalis (*Shan Yu Rou*), Semen Psoraleae Coryliflorae (*Bu Gu Zhi*), Fructus Lycii Chinensis (*Gou Qi Zi*), Semen Cuscutae (*Tu Si Zi*), Herba Cistanchis (*Rou Cong Rong*), Radix Morindae Officinalis (*Ba Ji Tian*), Radix Panacis Ginseng (*Ren Shen*), Rhizoma Atractylodis Macrocephelae (*Bai Zhu*), Placenta Hominis (*Ze He Che*), Colla Cornu Cervi (*Lu Jiao Jiao*), Fructus Schizandrae Chinensis (*Wu Wei Zi*), Fructus Foeniculi Vulgaris (*Xiao Hui Xiang*), and Semen Juglandis Regiae (*Hu Tao Ren*).

Ban Long Er Zhi Bai Bu Wan*:** This is a secret prescription. It is used to secure the root and safeguard the source, generate the essence and nourish the blood. It shores up and returns the heavenly true for major supplementation of vacuity detriment. [Ban Long Er Zhi Bai Bu Wan***] strengthens the source yang [in order to sire] many heirs, and long term administration is very effective in treating impotence. It is composed of Colla Cornu Cervi (*Lu Jiao Jiao*), Rhizoma Polygonati (*Huang Jing*), Fructus Lycii Chinensis (*Gou Qi Zi*), Radix Coquitus Rehmanniae (*Shu Di*), Semen Cuscutae (*Tu Si Zi*), Fructus Rosae Laevigatae (*Jin Ying Zi*), Tuber Ophiopogonis Japonicae (*Mai Men Dong*), Tuber Asparagi Cochinensis (*Tian Men Dong*), Radix Achyranthis Bidentatae (*Niu Xi*), Arillus Euphorbiae Longanae (*Long Yan Rou*), Cornu Degelatinum Cervi (*Lu Jiao Shuang*), Radix Panacis Ginseng (*Ren Shen*), Radix Astragali Seu Hedysari (*Huang Qi*), Sclerotium Poriae Cocoris (*Fu Ling*), Radix Dioscoreae Oppositae (*Shan Yao*), Fructus Corni Officinalis (*Shan Yu Rou*), Radix Anemarrhenae (*Zhi Mu*), and Fructus Schizandrae Chinensis (*Wu Wei Zi*).

3. Prescriptions for enriching and nourishing the kidney yin:

Liu Wei Di Huang Wan (available as a prepared medicine): This is *Shen Qi Wan* with the deletion of Radix Praeparatus Aconiti Carmichaeli (*Fu Zi*) and Cortex Cinnamomi (*Rou Gui*).

Zuo Gui Wan (available as a prepared medicine): *You Gui Wan* is primarily for supplementing the kidney yang, and *Zuo Gui Wan* is primarily for nourishing the kidney yin. It is composed of Radix Coquitus Rehmanniae (*Shu Di*), Radix Dioscoreae Oppositae (*Shan Yao*), Fructus Lycii Chinensis (*Gou Qi Zi*), Fructus Corni Officinalis (*Shan Yu Rou*), Radix Achyranthis Bidentatae (*Niu Xi*), Semen Cuscutae (*Tu Si Zi*), Cornu Degelatinum Cervi (*Lu Jiao Shuang*), and Plastrum Testudinis (*Gui Ban*). In the treatment of impotence *Zuo Gui Wan* is more effective than ***Liu Wei Di Huang Wan*.**

4. Prescriptions for simultaneously treating the heart and spleen:

Gui Pi Wan (available in prepared form): This prescription was used strictly by the medical factions of the Song Dynasty and plucked from the *Fu Ren Liang Fang*. It recognized this prescription as treating dual vacuity of heart and spleen. It is characterized by symptoms of an embarrassing nature, such as irregular menstruation in women. Therefore, this condition encompasses impotence. This prescription is presently used in illnesses related to blood patterns and patterns pertaining to neurological function but is also quite effective in treating impotence. It contains Radix Panacis Ginseng (*Ren Shen*), Radix Astragali Seu Hedysari (*Huang Qi*), Rhizoma Atractylodis Macrocephelae (*Bai Zhu*), Sclerotium Poriae Cocoris (*Fu Shen*), Semen Zizyphii Spinosae (*Suan Zao Ren*), Arillus Euphorbiae Longanae (*Lung Yan Rou*), Radix Polygalae Tenuifoliae (*Yuan Zhi*), Radix Saussureae Seu Vladimiriae (*Mu Xiang*), Radix Glycyrrhizae (*Gan Cao*), Rhizoma Desiccata Zingiberis (*Gan Jiang*), and Fructus Zizyphi Jujubae (*Da Zao*).

5. Prescriptions for clearing and transforming dampness and heat:

***Dao Chi San*:** This well known prescription is by the famous Qian Yi of the Song Dynasty and is composed of Radix Coquitus Rehmanniae (*Shu Di*), Caulis Bambusae In Taeniis (*Zhu Ru*), Caulis Akebiae Mutong (*Mu Tong*), and Radix Glycyrrhizae (*Gan Cao*). The formula addresses heart fire entering the small intestine and thus is employed to clear heat and disinhibit dampness.

Zi Shen Wan (available as a prepared medication): This prescription is the creation of Li Dong [yuan] of the Jin/Yuan Dynasties. It contains the three ingredients, Radix Anemarrhenae (*Zhi Mu*), Cortex Phellodendri (*Huang Bo*), and Cortex Cinnamomi (*Rou Gui*). It is quite appropriate for use in cases of impotence with urinary frequency or urinary inhibition.

Gan Lu Xiao Du Dan (available as a prepared medication): This prescription is the creation of the Qing Dynasty specialist in warm illnesses, Wang Meng-ying. It is composed of Herba Agastachis Seu Pogostemi (*Huo Xiang*), Semen Dolichoris Lablabis (*Bian Dou*), Rhizoma Acori Graminei (*Shi Chang Pu*), Herba Artemesiae Capillaris (*Yin Chen Hao*), Talcum (*Hua Shi*), Caulis Akebiae Mutong (*Mu Tong*), Radix Scutellariae Baicalensis (*Huang Qin*), Fructus Forsythiae Suspensae (*Lian Qiao*), Herba Menthae (*Bo He*), Rhizoma Belamcandae (*She Gan*), and Bulbus Fritillariae Thunbergii (*Bei Mu*). Today this prescription has an exceedingly wide range of uses and is used to good effect in the treatment of damp heat impotence as well.

6. Prescriptions for coursing the liver and resolving depression:

Xiao Yao Wan (available as a prepared medicine): Called *Xiao Yao* [free and easy] powder, the implication is that, after administration of this prescription, the patient's emotions will feel relaxed and the liver qi will become ordered. This is a prescription from our nation's Song dynasty issued as a prepared medication. It is composed of Radix Bupleuri (*Chai Hu*), Rhizoma Atractylodis Macrocephelae (*Bai Zhu*), Radix Angelicae Sinensis (*Dang Gui*), Radix Albus Paeoniae Lactiflorae (*Bai Shao*), Herba Menthae (*Bo He*), Sclerotium Poriae Cocoris (*Fu Ling*), and Radix Glycyrrhizae (*Gan Cao*).

***Miao Xiang San*:** This is a standard prescription from the Song Dynasty composed of Cinnabaris (*Zhu Sha*), Sclerotium Pararadicis Poriae Cocoris (*Fu Shen*), Radix Polygalae Tenuifoliae (*Yuan Zhi*), Radix Platycodi Grandiflorae (*Jie Geng*), Radix Saussureae Seu Vladimiriae (*Mu Xiang*), Secretio Moschi Moschiferi (*She Xiang*), Radix Panacis Ginseng (*Ren Shen*), Radix Astragali Seu Hedysari (*Huang Qi*), Radix Dioscoreae Oppositae (*Shan Yao*), and Radix Glycyrrhizae (*Gan Cao*).

In modern times there has been a great deal of clinical fumbling about [in the search for new medicines] within the medical specialties, and a large number of experiential prescriptions have been created for the treatment of impotence. There are a large number of new medicines in the herb shops as well. All of these medications should be employed based on the constitutional situation of the individual in order to achieve the best results.

Cases

Dual vacuity of heart and spleen. [VII]

Gao, a 25 year old farmer, was diagnosed on July 4th, 1981. He was married and had been having sexual relations for two years. However, he was so nervous that he would have an emission even before he became fully erect. In seeking medical advice, he had tried every means possible but to no avail.

Diagnostic examination: Both his body and spirit were fatigued. He suffered from heart vexation, insomnia, palpitations, little appetite, and a dull facial complexion. His tongue had little moss and a slightly red tip, while his pulse was floating, empty, and weak in the cubit position.

This pattern pertained to a dual vacuity of heart and spleen as well as a failure of the kidney to contain the essence. The indicated treatment was aimed at supplementing and boosting the heart and spleen, settling the heart and assimilating the kidney.

Prescription:

Rhizoma Atractylodis Macrocephelae (*Bai Zhu*) 10g
Radix Astragali Seu Hedysari (*Huang Qi*) 20g
Sclerotium Pararadicis Poriae Cocoris (*Fu Shen*) 15g
Radix Codonopsis Pilosulae (*Dang Shen*) 20g
Radix Polygalae Tenuifoliae (*Yuan Zhi*) 6g
Semen Zizyphi Spinosae (*Suan Zao Ren*) 20g
Radix Saussureae Seu Vladimiriae (*Mu Xiang*) 6g
Arillus Longanae Euphorbiae (*Long Yan Rou*) 20g
Radix Angelicae Sinensis (*Dang Gui*) 10g
Ootheca Mantidis (*Sang Piao Xiao*) 12g
Os Draconis (*Long Gu*) 30g
Concha Ostreae (*Mu Li*) 30g
Rhizoma Coptidis Chinensis (*Huang Lian*) 1.5g
Cortex Cinnamomi (*Rou Gui*) 3g
Radix Glycyrrhizae (*Gan Cao*) 6g

The patient was urged to temporarily regulate his desires as if there were a curtain between himself and a distant relation [*i.e.*, totally abstain from sexual activity].

[The patient's] premature ejaculation and impotence diminished slightly following four *ji* [formulas] of the above prescription. With administration of ten more *ji*, all his symptoms diminished. His medication was switched to a pill format and, sure enough, with administration of this, a positive outcome was obtained. His wife gave birth in October of 1982.

Vacuity of kidney yang

Wei, a 38 year old male, was first diagnosed September 14, 1978. He had noticed an overall lack of strength in the past three weeks with cephalic clouding, somnolence, an occasional sense of thoracic oppression, and shortness of breath. Of late, he had been particularly afraid of chilling winds. His back and knees were sore, his urination was shortened and frequent, and his libido had recently declined (such that, if his wife did not initiate sex, neither would he). When he did have sex, his erection was poor and he would quickly spend his essence. His tongue coat was thin and white, while his pulse was thin and frail. The pattern pertained to a vacuity of kidney yang and a failure of securing and assimilation. Treatment was indicated to warm the kidney and absorb the qi, secure the kidney and astringe the essence.

Prescription:

Cortex Cinnamomi (*Rou Gui*) 10g
Radix Praeparatus Aconiti Carmichaeli (*Fu Zi*) 15g (decocted previously)
Cortex Eucommiae (*Du Zhong*) 20g

Fructus Rosae Laevigatae (*Jin Ying Zi*) 20g
Cornu Degelatinum Cervi (*Lu Jiao Shuang*) 10g (dissolved)
Radix Coquitus Rehmanniae (*Shu Di*) 20g
Radix Dioscoreae Oppositae (*Shan Yao*) 20g
Rhizoma Curculiginis Orchoidis (*Xian Mao*) 20g
Herba Epimedii (*Yin Yang Huo*) 20g
Fructus Corni Officinalis (*Shan Yu Rou*) 20g
Semen Euryalis Ferocis (*Qian Shi*) 20g
Herba Cistanchis (*Rou Cong Rong*) 12g
Fructus Lycii Chinensis (*Gou Qi Zi*) 12g
Sclerotium Poriae Cocoris (*Fu Ling*) 12g
Fructus Schizandrae Chinensis (*Wu Wei Zi*) 12g

This was decocted in water and administered twice daily. Following administration of five *ji* [formulas], all the symptoms had diminished somewhat. With continuous administration of another ten *ji,* his spirit essence markedly improved, as did his libido. The premature ejaculation, however, persisted. He was instructed to eat crow, turtle, and black male chicken as well as moderate his sexual activity. Having recuperated over a period of six months, his sexual function returned to normal. On a follow-up visit in 1983, he reported no recurrence of the premature ejaculation and was pronounced completely cured.

Vacuity of yin and harassment of fire

Zhang, a 29 year old male, was diagnosed on April 16th, 1978. He had developed premature ejaculation after having been married and tended to cephalic dizziness and heat in the centers of the hands and feet. He suffered from overall weakness in his body, lumbar soreness and limpness. His tongue body was red with a yellow and white moss, and his pulse was wiry and rapid.

[The pattern pertained to a vacuity of yin and a harassment of fire.]

Prescription:

Radix Coquitus Rehmanniae (*Shu Di*) 25g
Radix Dioscoreae Oppositae (*Shan Yao*) 25g
Fructus Ligustri Lucidi (*Nu Zhen Zi*) 20g
Semen Astragali (*Sha Yuan Ji Li*) 20g
Semen Euryalis Ferocis (*Qian Shi*) 20g
Fructus Rosae Laevigatae (*Jin Ying Zi*) 20g
Semen Nelumbinis Nuciferae (*Lian Zi*) 15g
Fructus Schizandrae Chinensis (*Wu Wei Zi*) 15g
Herba Ecliptae Prostratae (*Han Lian Cao*) 15g
Cortex Phellodendri (*Huang Bo*) 10g
Radix Anemarrhenae (*Zhi Mu*) 10g

Decocted in water.

Following administration of 15 of the above formula, all the symptoms disappeared and his premature ejaculation was corrected. During a follow-up visit 18 months later, he reported that his wife was four months pregnant.

Vacuity of heart and kidney

Tian, a 40 year old office worker, was first diagnosed in July, 1984. Over the course of the previous year the patient had suffered from soreness and limpness in his lumbar spine as well as urgent pain. His entire body lacked strength; there was fatigue and a sense of lassitude. All these symptoms became more obvious when engaging in sexual activity, and he slept little at night and dreamt a great deal. He had taken Western medications, but they had had no positive effect. In recent months, he had developed palpitations, flusteredness, and a tendency to become easily frightened. Each time he would have sex, he would barely get [his penis] inserted [into the vagina] and he would spend. This would be followed by soreness and limpness and he could never complete the sexual activity. Relations with his wife were, therefore, not harmonious and this person's mood was that of shouldering a heavy burden. His tongue was pale white and his pulse was wiry and fine. This pattern pertained to a vacuity of heart and kidney qi and a loss of the kidney's capacity for storage. The essence gate was not secure and, thus, there was premature ejaculation. Treatment measures were indicated to nourish the heart and calm the spirit and supplement the kidney's capacity to store the essence.

Prescription:

Radix Coquitus Rehmanniae (*Shu Di*) 20g
Radix Codonopsis Pilosulae (*Dang Shen*) 20g
Fructus Lycii Chinensis (*Gou Qi Zi*) 25g
Semen Biotae Officinalis (*Bai Zi Ren*) 15g
Fructus Schizandrae Chinensis (*Wu Wei Zi*) 15g
Fructus Corni Officinalis (*Shan Yu Rou*) 15g
Sclerotium Pararadicis Poriae Cocoris (*Fu Shen*) 15g
Radix Dioscoreae Oppositae (*Shan Yao*) 15g
Radix Angelicae Sinensis (*Dang Gui*) 15g
Semen Euryalis Ferocis (*Qian Shi*) 15g
Semen Cnidii Monierii (*She Chuang Zi*) 15g
Rhizoma Cistanchis (*Rou Cong Rong*) 15g

Decocted in water.

With continued administration of ten *ji* of this formula, all the symptoms improved. The medication was later switched to pill form, and, with two months of continuous administration, he was completely cured.

Wang Qi

Depressive stasis of liver qi

The patient was a 24 year old male. He had been a habitual masturbator in his youth. Three months previously, he had gotten married and discovered that he was impotent. His testicles were damp and chilled and he suffered from occasional seminal efflux. His face was emaciated and he was pessimistic. He had a thin, white tongue coat, and his pulse was slightly wiry. His thoughts were disordered and scattered; the ancestral sinew was extremely tense and not functioning at all. He simultaneously experienced seminal efflux which was attributed to a disorder of the liver and kidney.

The therapy indicated was that of coursing the liver and soothing depression, enriching water and moistening wood. [These measures were] assisted by measures for unblocking the collaterals. ***Si Ni San*** together with modified ***San Cai Feng Sui Dan*** was administered.

Radix Bupleuri (*Chai Hu*) 12g
Radix Albus Paeoniae Lactiflorae (*Bai Shao*) 10g
Fructus Citri Seu Ponciri (*Zhi Ke*) 6g
Radix Glycyrrhizae (*Gan Cao*) 6g
Tuber Ophiopogonis Japonicae (*Mai Men Dong*) 10g
Radix Coquitus Rehmanniae (*Shu Di*) 15g
Radix Pseudostellariae Heterophyllae (*Tai Zi Shen*) 15g
Scolopendra Subspinipes (*Wu Gong*) 2g
Fructus Seu Semen Amomi (*Sha Ren*) 3g
Radix Phellodendri (*Huang Bo*) 6g

The patient reported that following seven doses of the medication the damp chill in the testicles had diminished. He was able to achieve an erection, albeit only for a short time, and was not inclined toward anything too daring. His tongue coat was slimy and so Semen Plantaginis (*Che Qian Zi*) and Semen Vaccariae Segetalis (*Wang Bu Liu Xing*) were added to the original prescription to transform dampness and circulate stasis, and his impotence was ultimately cured.

Wu Jin-zeng

A case of phlegm and stasis obstructing the collaterals

Jie was a 28 year old worker. He became impotent after having gotten married, and they had been living together as man and wife for three years without having conceived. He suffered from lumbar soreness, cephalic dizziness, low libido, inability to maintain an erection, and unsuccessful intercourse. Nevertheless, he would occasionally experience a spontaneous erection while sleeping. He was first diagnosed on January 5th, 1983 and administered ***Ma Qian Tong Guan San*** with the addition of 18 grams of Nidus Vespae (*Lu Feng Fang*) which was powdered and administered for 40 days. With a single therapeutic course [40 days], he was able to achieve an erection, although he could not maintain it for long. [The patient] continued administration of the above medication combined with administration of 0.6 grams of aged tortoise (*Gui Ling Ji*) each day. He completed two courses of the medication and was able to sustain an erection as well as twice having successful intercourse. The plan was to gradually decrease the dosage of the medication [by taking one dose per day] in order to consolidate the therapeutic effect.

During a follow-up visit on March 17th, 1984, he reported that he no longer suffered from impotence and that his wife had been pregnant for over two months.

Prescription:

prepared Semen Strychnotis (*Ma Qian Zi*) 12g
raw Herba Ephedrae (*Ma Huang*) 12g
Rhizoma Acori Graminei (*Shi Chang Pu*) 12g
Scolopendra Subspinipes (*Wu Gong*) 18g
Radix Angelicae Sinensis (*Dang Gui*) 60g
Radix Albus Paeoniae Lactiflorae (*Bai Shao*) 60g
raw Radix Glycyrrhizae (*Gan Cao*) 60g

This was ground into a fine powder.

To this was added Nidus Vespae (*Lu Feng Fang*) 18g, also ground into a powder. The [entire preparation was] divided into 40 envelopes. One envelope was taken nightly with wine. Forty days constituted a therapeutic course.

Comment: In this pattern, the essential pathodynamic was that of phlegm, stagnation, and fire. Therefore ***Ma Qian Tong Guan San*** was employed as the primary therapeutic prescription. Semen Strychnotis has a bitter taste and cold nature. It promotes free flow of the collaterals and is an important medicinal for dispersing blood heat. The alkalines within Semen Strychnotis contain wood tortoise alkalines [strychnine]. These stimulate the central nervous system, and, particularly in the spinal chord, exhibit a high degree of selectivity in their capacity to heighten the excitability of the ejaculatory centers. This medicinal is, however, definitely toxic, and the standards used in its processing must be rigorously controlled. If sensations of contracture of the flesh occur following administration of this medicinal, its use should be discontinued. Rhizoma Acori Graminei functions to transform turbidity and open the orifices. Herba Ephedrae has a sweet and warm nature and opens the nine orifices. Of Scolopendra Subspinipes Zhang Xi-chun states that it:

> . . .is known for its capacity to rapidly travel internally to the viscera and bowels as well as externally to the connecting channels. It functions to open up all the locations of qi and blood congestion.

Rhizoma Acori Graminei functions to transform turbidity and open the orifices. According to the *Tang Ben Cao*, Nidus Vespae, when "charred and administered with wine, governs impotence". These medicinals are assisted by Radix Angelicae Sinensis, which nourishes and quickens the blood, Radix Albus Paeoniae Lactiflorae, which supplements and softens the liver and brightens and nourishes the ancestral sinew, and Radix Glycyrrhizae, which harmonizes the middle and resolves toxicity. It [Radix Glycyrrhizae] oversees the tendency of Herba Ephedrae to injure the yin, and in this, they supplement and compliment each other.

Lin Hong-yi

A case of fright injuring the kidneys

Sheng, a 28 year old farmer, was habitually frightened and quite suspicious. He had been out and about amusing himself during a national celebration till around midnight when he headed for home. He was riding his bicycle carelessly down a hill when he tumbled off. He was then terrified when a neighbor's dog violently attacked him. The affair was over, but he began experiencing spermatorrhea which would dampen the inside of his trousers. Afterward, he became impotent, his heart essence was repressed, it was difficult for him to sleep at night, and he suffered from palpitations. His tongue was pale with a thin white coat, and his pulse was fine and wiry, lacking strength. ***Da Bu Yuan Jian*** and modified ***Gui Pi Tang*** were prescribed:

Radix Coquitus Rehmanniae (*Shu Di*) 20g
Fructus Corni Officinalis (*Shan Yu Rou*) 10g
Radix Dioscoreae Oppositae (*Shan Yao*) 10g
Fructus Lycii Chinensis (*Gou Qi Zi*) 30g
Cortex Eucommiae Ulmoides (*Du Zhong*) 15g
Radix Codonopsis Pilosulae (*Dang Shen*) 30g
Radix Praeparatus Glycyrrhizae (*Zhi Gan Cao*) 6g
Radix Astragali Seu Hedysari (*Huang Qi*) 30g
Arillus Longanae Euphorbiae (*Long Yan Rou*) 30g
Sclerotium Paradicis Poriae Cocoris (*Fu Shen*) 10g
Radix Saussureae Seu Vladimiriae (*Mu Xiang*) 3g
Semen Zizyphi Spinosae (*Suan Zao Ren*) 30g
Radix Polygalae Tenuifoliae (*Yuan Zhi*) 10g

14 *ji* were administered in decoction.

Comment: The "*Yang Wei Pian*" of *Jing Yue Quan Shu* states that all cases of unexplainable fright will also result in impotence. The classic states that fright damages the kidneys, and so we can say that this patient was habitually frightened as a consequence of a sudden scare. He suffered spermatorrhea, his spirit was scattered, his kidneys were damaged, and he became impotent. Therapy began with the heart and kidneys and proceeded with [measures for] settling the spirit and securing the kidney qi. He achieved a complete cure after ten doses.

Impotence due to dampness and heat in the *yang ming*

Zhou, a 24 year old commune member, had been impotent for one year. He had taken medicinal substances to supplement the yang, such as the folk prescription ***Bing Suan Luan Wan Su***, but there had been no positive changes in his condition. His urine was yellow and hot and, moreover, there was dribbling and a sense of incomplete [urination]. Examination of his tongue revealed that it was slightly red with a white, somewhat thick, pasty coat. His lips and mouth were dry and his pulse was rapid. His body was fat and strong. This condition was one of an exuberance of *yang ming* heat and deep-lying fire in the spleen channel. This manifested concurrently with dampness and heat in the urinary bladder and a slackening of the ancestral sinew, resulting in inability to produce an erection. This is the meaning of [the statement], "in treating impotence treat only the *yang ming*". The plan was to employ formulas for clearing and disinhibiting the dampness and heat in the middle and lower warmers and draining the repletion heat in the spleen channel.

Herba Dendrobii (*Shi Hu*) 20g
Semen Coicis Lachryma-jobi (*Yi Yi Ren*) 30g
Caulis Bambusae In Taeniis (*Zhu Ru*) 30g
Rhizoma Alismatis (*Ze Xie*) 10g
Herba Eupatorii Fortunei (*Pei Lan*) 10g
Apex Rhizomatis Coptidis Chinensis (*Huang Lian Wei*) 10g
Fructus Trichosanthis Kirlowii (*Gua Lou*) 10g
Radix Trichosanthes Kirlowii (*Tian Hua Fen*) 10g
Radix Ledebouriellae Sesloidis (*Fang Feng*) 10g
Pericarpium Citri Reticulatae (*Chen Pi*) 10g
Radix Achyranthis Bidentatae (*Niu Xi*) 10g
Cortex Phellodendri (*Huang Bo*) 10g
Rhizoma Atractylodis (*Cang Zhu*) 12g
Radix Glycyrrhizae (*Gan Cao*) 5g

Decocted in water and divided into two doses daily.

After administration of 12 of the above formula, the dryness of the patient's lips was noticeably relieved, the burning urination had diminished somewhat, and his sexual function had improved a little. His tongue body was normal, his tongue coat was still white and a little thick, and his pulse was wiry and a little rapid. This pattern reflected a gradual clearing of the dampness and heat and an elimination of the deep-lying fire in the spleen channel. The Caulis Bambusae In Taeniis, Herba Eupatorii Fortunei, Apex Rhizoma Coptidis Chinensis, Fructus Trichosanthis Kirlowii, Radix Trichosanthis Kirlowii, and Radix Ledebouriellae Sesloidis were deleted from the previous prescription and Semen Nelumbinis Nuciferae 12g, Herba Cistanchis 12g, and Radix Dioscoreae Oppositae 15g, were added. With continued administration of 12 more prescriptions, he was able to maintain an erection which was firm and strong. His sexual vitality normalized, and there were no more recurrences [of his illness].

BIBLIOGRAPHY

I. Ming, *Yi Te Se Jing Yan Jing Hua Chen Zilin* and Song, *Zujing*, Shanghai College of Chinese Medicine Press, 1987

II. *Qian Jia Miao Fang*, Vol I and II, edited by Li Wen-liang & Qi Qiong et. al., Liberation Army Publishing, Beijing, 1985

III. *Qin Bo Wei Yi Wen Ji*, by Qin Bo-wei, Hunan Science & Technology Press, 1981

IV. *Shang Hai Lao Zhong Yi Jing Yan Shi Pian*, edited by the Shanghai Hygiene Bureau, published by Shanghai Science and Technology Press, 1978

V. *Zhong Jing Fang Zai Ji Nan Zhong Bing Zhong De Yun Yong*, edited by the Shanghai Chinese Medical Literature Legation, Shanghai College of TCM Press, 1987

VI. *Zhong Guo Xian Dai Ming Zhong Yi Yi An Jing Hua*, edited by Zhong Jian-hua et.al., Beijing Press, 1990

VII. *Zhong Guo Nan Ke Yi An Tian Jin*, Science and Technology Translation Press Corporation, 1990

VIII. *Nan Ke Zhong Zhi Xin Fa*, by Cheng, Wang, and Liu Beijing Science and Technology Press, 1991

IX. *Zhong Yi Nan Ke Bai Wen (100 Questions on TCM Urology)*, Wu Yin-geng & Shen Qing-fa, Shanghai Science & Technology Press, Shanghai, 1990

INDEX

D

E

F

G

H

I

J

K

L

M

N

O

P

U

V

W

X

Y

Z

OTHER BOOKS ON CHINESE MEDICINE AVAILABLE FROM BLUE POPPY PRESS

PMS: Its Cause, Diagnosis & Treatment According to Traditional Chinese Medicine by Bob Flaws ISBN 0-936185-22-8 $14.95

SOMETHING OLD, SOMETHING NEW; Essays on the TCM Description of Western Herbs, Pharmaceuticals, Vitamins & Minerals by Bob Flaws ISBN 0-936185-21-X $19.95

SCATOLOGY & THE GATE OF LIFE: The Role of the Large Intestine in Immunity, An Integrated Chinese-Western Approach by Bob Flaws ISBN 0-936185-20-1 $12.95

MENOPAUSE, A Second Spring: Making A Smooth Transition with Traditional Chinese Medicine by Honora Lee Wolfe ISBN 0-936185-18-X $14.95

MIGRAINES & TRADITIONAL CHINESE MEDICINE: A Layperson's Guide by Bob Flaws ISBN 0-936185-15-5 $11.95

STICKING TO THE POINT: A Rational Methodology for the Step by Step Administration of an Acupuncture Treatment by Bob Flaws ISBN 0-936185-17-1 $14.95

ENDOMETRIOSIS & INFERTILITY AND TRADITIONAL CHINESE MEDICINE: A Laywoman's Guide by Bob Flaws ISBN 0-936185-14-7 $9.95

THE BREAST CONNECTION: A Laywoman's Guide to the Treatment of Breast Disease by Chinese Medicine by Honora Lee Wolfe ISBN 0-936185-13-9 $8.95

NINE OUNCES: A Nine Part Program For The Prevention of AIDS in HIV Positive Persons by Bob Flaws ISBN 0-936185-12-0 $9.95

THE TREATMENT OF CANCER BY INTEGRATED CHINESE-WESTERN MEDICINE by Zhang Dai-zhao, trans. by Zhang Ting-liang ISBN 0-936185-11-2 $16.95

A HANDBOOK OF TRADITIONAL CHINESE DERMATOLOGY by Liang Jian-hui, trans. by Zhang Ting-liang & Bob Flaws, ISBN 0-936185-07-4 $14.95

A HANDBOOK OF TRADITIONAL CHINESE GYNECOLOGY by Zhejiang College of TCM, trans. by Zhang Ting-liang, ISBN 0-936185-06-6 (2nd edit.) $21.95

FREE & EASY: Traditional Chinese Gynecology for American Women 2nd Edition, by Bob Flaws, ISBN 0-936185-05-8 $15.95

PRINCE WEN HUI'S COOK: Chinese Dietary Therapy by Bob Flaws & Honora Lee Wolfe, ISBN 0-912111-05-4, $12.95 (Published by Paradigm Press, Brookline, MA)

THE DAO OF INCREASING LONGEVITY AND CONSERVING ONE'S LIFE by Anna Lin & Bob Flaws, ISBN 0-936185-24-4 $16.95

FIRE IN THE VALLEY: The TCM Diagnosis and Treatment of Vaginal Diseases by Bob Flaws ISBN 0-936185-25-2 $16.95

HIGHLIGHTS OF ANCIENT ACUPUNCTURE PRESCRIPTIONS trans. by Honora Lee Wolfe & Rose Crescenz ISBN 0-936185-23-6 $14.95

ARISAL OF THE CLEAR: A Simple Guide to Healthy Eating According to Traditional Chinese Medicine by Bob Flaws, ISBN #-936185-27-9 $8.95

CERVICAL DYSPLASIA & PROSTATE CANCER: HPV, A HIDDEN LINK? by Bob Flaws, ISBN 0-936185-19-8 $23.95

PEDIATRIC BRONCHITIS: ITS CAUSE, DIAGNOSIS & TREATMENT ACCORDING TO TRADITIONAL CHINESE MEDICINE trans. by Gao Yu-li and Bob Flaws, ISBN 0-936185-26-0 $15.95

AIDS & ITS TREATMENT ACCORDING TO TRADITIONAL CHINESE MEDICINE by Huang Bing-shan, trans. by Fu-Di & Bob Flaws, ISBN 0-936185-28-7 $24.95

ACUTE ABDOMINAL SYNDROMES: Their Diagnosis & Treatment by Combined Chinese-Western Medicine by Alon Marcus, ISBN 0-936185-31-7 $16.95

BEFORE COMPLETION: Essays on the Practice of TCM by Bob Flaws, ISBN 0-936185-32-5, $16.95

MY SISTER, THE MOON: The Diagnosis & Treatment of Menstrual Diseases by Traditional Chinese Medicine by Bob Flaws, ISBN 0-936185-34-1, $24.95

FU QING-ZHU'S GYNECOLOGY trans. by Yang Shou-zhong and Liu Da-wei, ISBN 0-936185-35-X, $21.95

FLESHING OUT THE BONES: The Importance of Case Histories in Chinese Medicine trans. by Charles Chace. ISBN 0-936185-30-9, $18.95

CLASSICAL MOXIBUSTION SKILLS IN CONTEMPORARY CLINICAL PRACTICE by Sung Baek, ISBN 0-936185-16-3 $10.95

THE MEDICAL I CHING: Oracle of the Healer Within by Miki Shima, OMD, ISBN 0-936185-38-4, $19.95

MASTER TONG'S ACUPUNCTURE: An Ancient Lineage for Modern Practice, trans. and commentary by Miriam Lee, OMD, ISBN 0-936185-37-6, $19.95

A HANDBOOK OF TCM UROLOGY & MALE SEXUAL DYSFUNCTION by Anna Lin, OMD, ISBN 0-936185-36-8, $16.95

Li Dong-yuan's TREATISE ON THE SPLEEN & STOMACH, A Translation of the *Pi Wei Lun* by Yang Shou-zhong & Li Jian-yong, ISBN 0-936185-41-4, $21.95

PATH OF PREGNANCY, VOL. I, Gestational Disorders by Bob Flaws, ISBN 0-936185-39-2, $16.95

PATH OF PREGNANCY, VOL. II, Postpartum Diseases by Bob Flaws, ISBN 0-936185-42-2, $18.95

How to Have a HEALTHY PREGNANCY, HEALTHY BIRTH with Traditional Chinese Medicine by Honora Lee Wolfe, ISBN 0-936185-40-6, $9.95

MASTER HUA'S CLASSIC OF THE CENTRAL VISCERA by Hua Tuo, translated by Yang Shou-zhong, ISBN 0-936185-43-0, $21.95

A NEW AMERICAN ACUPUNCTURE: Acupuncture Osteopathy, by Mark Seem, ISBN 0-936185-44-9, $19.95

THE HEART & ESSENCE OF DAN-XI'S METHODS OF TREATMENT by Zhu Dan-xi, trans. by Yang Shou-zhong. ISBN 0-936185-50-3, $21.95

HOW TO WRITE A TCM HERBAL FORMULA A Logical Methodology for the Formulation & Administration of Chinese Herbal Medicine in Decoction, by Bob Flaws, ISBN 0-936185-49-X, $10.95

FULFILLING THE ESSENCE: A Handbook of Traditional & Contemporary Chinese Treatments for Female Infertility by Bob Flaws. ISBN 0-936185-48-1, $19.95